Innovative Decision Making in Healthcare

Leslie Neal-Boylan • Steven Rotkoff

Innovative Decision Making in Healthcare

A Case-Based Approach
to Nursing Leadership
in Academic and Clinical Settings

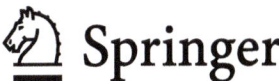 Springer

Leslie Neal-Boylan
Nursing
Mansfield Kaseman Health Clinic
Rockville, MD
USA

Steven Rotkoff
Lansing, KS
USA

ISBN 978-3-030-72647-8   ISBN 978-3-030-72648-5   (eBook)
https://doi.org/10.1007/978-3-030-72648-5

This Springer imprint is published by the registered company Springer Nature Switzerland AG
The registered company address is: Gewerbestrasse 11, 6330 Cham, Switzerland

To all the faculty and staff with whom I have worked in my academic career. Nursing faculty and support staff are amazing people and I have been honored to work with them.

I've met great and awful academic leaders from a variety of disciplines. They taught me everything I know about leadership – what to do and what not to do. I am grateful to them all. I hope Red Teaming makes the great leaders even better and the awful leaders think carefully about how they lead.
— *Leslie Neal-Boylan*

To Libby who makes all my achievements possible and to Jack who showed me it was OK to be a heretic inside the Army.
— *Steven Rotkoff*

Preface

This book was written by a brother and sister team. Colonel (Retired) Steve Rotkoff is a West Point Graduate with 26 years of active military service and 15 years as a senior civilian working for the military. In that time, he served in Bosnia, Kosovo, Iraq, and Afghanistan as well as Germany and Korea. He developed and led the Red Team education program for the Army during his 15 years as a senior civilian. The story of how Red Teaming came about and why it matters to the military is his story.

Leslie Neal-Boylan (nee Rotkoff) is a family nurse practitioner and former professor and dean of nursing. During her time as a leader in both clinical and academic settings, she frequently called Steve to discuss strategies for managing leadership challenges. Red Teaming offered innovative options to typical nursing leadership strategies. That is her story.

Large successful organizations only learn from failure. If everything is going well, there is a tendency not to challenge methods. It is only once things have gone radically wrong that a large successful organization starts to reexamine their methods and culture. Such an event was Operation Iraqi Freedom (OIF) for the US Army. Steve was the deputy for the Combined-2 (C2) of the Combined Forces Land Component Coalition or (CFLCC). CFLCC was the highest headquarters for all ground components (Army, Marines, and to a limited degree Special Operations Forces) operating in Iraq. The C2 (Combined Intelligence Staff lead) was a two-star general and the senior intelligence officer for CFLCC. Steve, a colonel at the time, was his deputy.

In that position, Steve was privy to all of the senior leader meetings, planning, and decision making associated with the conduct of the war from June of 2002 when the planning began through May of 2003 when President Bush declared victory.

What happened and how and why it happened led to the development of a Red Team education program in the Army in 2005. During the planning stages of the war, senior leaders embraced an analogy often used by Secretary of Defense Donald Rumsfeld. His analogy was that post-OIF Iraq would be a lot like post-WWII Germany. Saddam Hussein was an analog for Hitler and the Iraqi people would respond to Saddam's death or capture as the Germans had – i.e., rebuild the country into a prosperous one. The basis for this thinking was that like Germany pre-WWII, Iraq had an educated populace and in addition it had a wealth of natural resources. The Tigris and Euphrates are the Fertile Crescent, Iraq is rich in oil and natural gas, and before the war, the place for brain surgery or other high-tech industry in the Middle East was centered in Baghdad. Thus, the theory posited that with Saddam gone, the Iraqis, like the Germans after WWII, would pick themselves up, leverage their educated populace and resource rich country, and rebuild. Iraq would then serve as a bulwark against terrorism in the Middle East and help stabilize Afghanistan and serve as a deterrent to Iran. This idea was so widely accepted at senior levels that there was little initial planning for the post-combat requirements of Iraq. US policy before the war began was for our armed forces to stay in Iraq for less than a year.

This entire analogy was flawed in its conception. Unlike the Germans, the Iraqis were divided into several groups that shared few, if any, common interests or perspectives. There was a historic split between Sunni and Shia. This split was enmity filled based on religious, political, and socio-economic chasms between the two groups. This split was very much exacerbated and fueled by Iran. There was a split between Arab and Kurd, with the Kurds seeing themselves as independent people held hostage inside of an artificial Iraqi state. Exacerbating both splits were the neighboring states. Iran was a supporter and supplier of the Shia and had every intention of turning Iraq into a client state. Turkey wanted to eradicate the threat of a Kurdish state on its southern border. Saudi Arabia (not immediately adjacent to Iraq like Turkey and Iran) was invested in the Iraqi Sunni population. Pakistan harbored insurgents and sold arms to all bidders. This was not postwar Germany after WWII!

During the planning and staging period for OIF (June 2002–March 2003), the senior leaders met with a host of different kinds of people who knew a lot about Iraq. Steve was in most of those meetings. In every one of those meetings, whether they were with ex-patriot Imams, PhD-prepared experts with a deep understanding of Iraq, or local Americans who had lived in Kuwait and studied the region (i.e., CIA or State Department folks), they universally told us that the analogy we accepted was wrong, explaining in detail the reasons described above.

One of those we interviewed said, "this will not be post WWII Germany, this will look like post Tito Yugoslavia but on steroids, everyone will be killing everyone." One of those we spoke to informed us that if we were going to invade Iraq and topple Saddam we needed to be prepared to have an active military presence in Iraq for 60 years. He said it would take two generations to stabilize Iraq in such a way as it could help stabilize the region. These comments reflect the general feedback of those who knew Iraq well.

Despite these misgivings, planning went along without consideration of the insights provided by those who knew Iraq well. In the aftermath, the haunting question was: "Why had we not listened to the repeated warnings given to us by the people who knew the country and people best?"

Steve led the Army Intelligence lessons learned group that formed in 2004–2005 to study why things had turned out differently than expected after Saddam fell. The first instinct of any organization that fails is to claim they did not have the information they needed to be successful.

Intelligence professionals are enamored with data. "If only we had all of the data, we would make the right decision," represents the philosophy underlying most intelligence thinking. This is patently untrue in general. For a moment, think of a chess match. Is any data hidden from either side? If not, why doesn't every match end in a draw? Because chess even at the most skilled level, like all decision making, is about more than simply data. It is about the opponent, understanding how he or she plays, tricking them into believing things they already want to believe so they fall into a trap, etc. This data centric way of thinking was clearly flawed based on our experience running up to Operation Iraqi Freedom (OIF).

Steve attempted to understand why the military did not listen, and began to encounter well-established decision-making biases, which, despite all his time as a leader, had never been included in his training. In the case of Iraq, everyone suffered from "ignoring disconfirming evidence." This bias is one where the group having thought deeply about a problem is confronted with new information that challenges their understanding of the problem and way forward.

When this happens, the team has two choices. The first is to step back and reconsider the problem in light of the new information. This is hard to do. It may invalidate the work done to date. The group believes it understood the issue prior to learning the new information and does not want to acknowledge these new data. This leads to the second choice to simply ignore the information and stay with the current perspective on the problem. That is what happened in Iraq.

This realization then raised the question, "how do we prevent this from happening again?" If the errors in judgment were not a result of lacking data – what was the cause? It was clear that four fundamental shortfalls in our planning process needed to be addressed:

1. To find ways to be more divergent in initial thinking
2. To foster empathy for those outside our own cultural experience
3. To find ways to mitigate groupthink
4. To introduce tools designed to foster considerations of alternative futures

As a consequence, the Army decided to change the decision-making culture by building a school designed to teach these methods to soldiers. The program was a great success evidenced by the fact that several of the tools we will discuss in this book have become part of Army doctrine and are now taught to leaders at every level. Additionally, Red Team tools and methods have been used in planning processes by the military on multiple occasions to address topics as diverse as combating ISIS to fighting Ebola.

Unlike many planning and decision-making methodologies Red Team methods are not a step by step process, like Lean or Six Sigma. Unfortunately, in many cases procedural step by step processes frequently lead to the completion of the process as the overriding objective, instead of improving the decision-making process. Many of the mistakes made by the military were a direct result of the fixation on the seven step Military Decision-Making Process (MDMP), interfering with versus enabling better thinking. MDMP is a well-respected method adopted by many other organizations as well as several militaries around the world. It is important to understand the army did not adopt Red Teaming because it had no decision- making process. It adopted it because it had such a thorough process that the process itself created a false sense of confidence in the decisions that were made. Additionally, the process is based on a very clear definition of the problem to be solved (the mission) and is constraining when faced with a complex problem such as in Iraq.

The steps of this process are as follows:

1. **Receipt of Mission** – This is when the higher headquarters tells you what to do. This works very well at a tactical level. The mission CFLCC was given was to defeat Saddam's forces and occupy the country. In retrospect that was the wrong mission. Our mission should have been to defeat Saddam and create conditions for a peaceful transition to power for a post Saddam government, of which the national command group should have provided some vision. However, since the WWII analogy was so embraced, the ascension of some post Saddam government was assumed as being peaceful and organic, despite all the feedback we received to the contrary. The problem with process, step by step planning, is that if you get the first step wrong, all of the rest becomes invalid.

2. **Mission Analysis** – This occurs when the subordinate unit takes the mission received in step one and considers the operational environment affecting the completion of that mission. It is integral to examine the environment or conditions needed to make the mission succeed.

3. **Course of Action Development** – This step includes a set of alternative approaches developed to accomplish the mission within the constraints revealed during the mission analysis. To use the "take a hill" analogy. At a minimum there are three ways to take the hill. Weight the attacking forces on the east (this assumes the unit is attacking south to north), weight the attacking forces on the west, or conduct a balanced attack. The advantages or disadvantages of each is based on the terrain, lines of sight, and other factors. In addition, the mix of forces can be varied to create different courses of action, armor heavy, infantry heavy, use of airborne, etc. The object of each course of action is to accomplish the mission received in step 1, with a full cognizance of the conditions explored in step 2.

4. **Course of Action Analysis** – This step occurs when each course of action is tested through a process of analysis. The operations officer and staff execute the course of action in a wargame. These can be highly sophisticated and digital, or they can be a simple sand table. The intelligence officer plays the enemy during the war game and tries to replicate enemy actions in response to the course of action being tested. There is always an assigned scribe who captures the thinking and actions of both sides. Of key importance during the preparation for Operation

Iraqi Freedom the wargames ended at CFLCCs successful occupation of Baghdad and the defeat of the Iraqi army. The post combat challenges of Iraq were never examined because they were never part of the mission!

5. *Course of Action Comparison* – Following the analysis, the different courses of action are compared to each other using a group of common metrics. These metrics might include: speed (how quickly did we accomplish the mission), expected casualties (again based on the wargame), post mission accomplishment posture (does one course of action leave us in a better position for the expected follow-on mission), ease of logistic support, etc. Each course of action is evaluated and given a score based on these common metrics. At the end of this phase there is usually a course of action that is most favored.

6. *Course of Action Approval* – At this stage, the planning team briefs the senior leader. The staff walks the leaders through each of the previously described steps. In a good unit, this results in a lot of cross talk among the leadership. Usually this is focused on the wargame, the metrics for evaluation, and the design of the most favored course of action. Usually, the decision coming out of these discussions is some variant of the most favored course of action, fine-tuned based on the collective experience of the leaders in the room.

7. *Orders Production* – After the senior leader has decided on the course of action, everyone must be informed of their responsibilities to make the action take place.

The Red Team approach is by design entirely different. The process comes down to five steps:

1. Spend time **understanding the root problem**, instead of the symptoms of the problem. This helps ensure the mission addresses the right problem.
2. Understand the time available for the Red Team, the audience for the Red Team, the people who will compose the Red Team, and the **circumstances under which the Red Team will be conducted**.
3. *Pick those tools most suited to that SPECIFIC circumstance.*
4. *Red Team*
5. *Present the results*

The analogy used around the use of Red Team tools is best compared to a golfer playing a hole. The golfer has a number of different clubs in his/her bag. Some they use frequently, some infrequently. The use of the right club in the right situation, along with the skill level of the golfer in using that club are the determinants of success. The longer the golfer practices with the tools (clubs) in different situations the more adept they become. This is the same for Red Team tools and methods.

While the military may seem vastly different from nursing, on closer scrutiny, decision making in nursing is not as different as it might first appear. Let's compare the MDMP model to the average school of nursing.

1. *Receipt of Mission* – Recall that in military organizations, this is the higher headquarters telling you what to do. In the case of an independent school or

college of nursing, the dean assigns the mission. In a department of nursing, the chair of the nursing department might receive the mission from a non-nursing dean. Like the military example, if the mission or charge is to revise the curriculum, the message is clear. However, if there has been no thought put into why the curriculum needs to be changed, such as increasing tuition, meeting a need in the community, or complying with professional standards, we might embark on a lengthy process that does not attract students or solve a problem, or align with advances in nursing. We will have wasted precious faculty and staff time because we didn't consider all options or include all pertinent voices.

2. *Mission Analysis* – For the military, this is where the subordinate unit considers the operational environment affecting the completion of that mission. Applying curriculum revision to this second step requires us to consider whether the school or department has the expertise to redesign the curriculum and teach the classes. How many students will be needed to bring in sufficient revenue to meet costs and then some? Will additional supplies, equipment, classroom space, clinical assignments, or classroom space be needed? What added value will the new curriculum bring to students and graduates? What do employers want in graduates from our programs?

3. *Course of Action Development* – This step is where a set of alternative approaches are developed to accomplish the mission within the constraints revealed during the mission analysis. How will the school or department proceed with planning and implementing the curriculum revision? Faculty are so busy, is there sufficient funding to hire a curriculum consultant to do the bulk of the work? If not, how can the timeline be developed to allow for frequent meetings? Who should attend the meetings? What is the university's process for approving the changes after the school or department develops them? The curriculum approval process timeline must be considered when deciding on the best approach.

4. *Course of Action Analysis* – For the military, this step is where each course of action is tested through a process of war gaming. In an academic setting, the dean or department chair might meet with key leaders to lay out proposed timelines and approaches.

5. *Course of Action Comparison* – The next step is to compare the different courses of action using a group of common metrics. These metrics might include *speed* (how quickly can we accomplish the mission according to each proposed timeline?), *potential problems* based in our action analysis, *post mission accomplishment posture* (will one course of action better enable us to move the new curriculum through the frequently cumbersome university curriculum approval process more quickly or be more likely to please university administrators because it will bring in more revenue?), *ease of support* (will faculty buy in to the need for a new curriculum? Will administration provide advance funding until the new curriculum can support itself?).

6. *Course of Action Approval* – During this stage, the planning team briefs the senior leaders of the unit. In our nursing education scenario, the dean or department chair consults their supervisor about the proposed curriculum revision.

7. ***Orders Production*** – Once the dean or department chair's supervisor approves the curriculum revision plan and timeline, the plan is shared with all nursing faculty and staff. Unlike in the military, faculty must have final say as faculty have responsibility for the curriculum. This is why it's vital to have key faculty with curriculum expertise involved in the early discussions and planning stages.

However, like the military, these processes can blind us to the underlying problem. If the mission as laid out by the nursing dean is flawed, then all subsequent actions are also flawed. How then do we have a conversation about the relevance of the initial mission and how do we include under-heard voices during the rest of the process? Red Teaming is the best approach.

Rockville, MD, USA   Leslie Neal-Boylan
Lansing, KS, USA   Steven Rotkoff

Acknowledgments

We gratefully acknowledge the incredible skill and talent of Ms. Tara Neal for her illustrations in this book. Much more of her work can be found at: https://www.pinterest.com/tara_w_neal/

— Leslie Neal-Boylan

My journey in Red Teaming would have never been possible without all of the following people: MG (RET) Spider Marks, COL (RET) Greg Fontenot, COL (RET) Maxie McFarland, Ori Brafman Lisa Kimball, Judah Pollack, GEN (RET) Keith Alexander, LTG (RET) Kimmons, GEN (RET) Bob Brown, and Whitney Hischier. Each of them either was a critical advocate that enabled Red Teaming to prosper or was a direct influence on how I thought about building better conversations and plans through the use of Red Team tools.

— Steven Rotkoff

How to Use This Book

The phrase Red Teaming is really a shorthand for learning to think, listen, and communicate in a new way. It is truly a meta-concept. People and organizations that use Red Teaming understand that all but the most simple and routine problems are deserving of thoughtful consideration. They know that alternative perspectives and truth telling by subordinates to seniors are critical for informed decisions. They understand that the future "has a mind of its own" and will almost always turn out differently than anticipated. The tools and methods introduced in this book are merely a way of opening up the reader to these important concepts. These tools are not all encompassing. Once you learn to think like a Red Teamer you will tailor them or build your own for whatever specific purpose you need.

You will not be perfect at implementing these ideas on the first try. Using Red Team methods is much like learning a new language. It will take some practice to get good at it, but once you are comfortable you will begin to think in that new language. Do not feel compelled to use (or even like) all of the tools about which you will read. A good Red Teamer generally has 6–10 tools they use all of the time and a handful they use on occasion. That set of preferred tools are different for each Red Teamer and reflect the Zen notion that no person crosses the same river twice – the second time, the river has changed and the person has changed. So too, the right mix of tools depends upon the skills and comfort level of the person using them. The good news is that even a flawed attempt at using these tools is better than no attempt at using them.

Embracing the ideas that divergence of thought should proceed convergence on an action plan, that everyone should be heard, that the quality of an idea should be judged independent of the source of the idea, and the future may well turn out differently despite our best efforts to plan will all improve the quality of the decisions made by the group.

The book is organized into introductory chapters followed by cases. The introductory chapters explain the Red Teaming approach in detail and the cases illustrate how to apply the approach and the tools to situations in academic and clinical settings. This book was written during the COVID-19 pandemic. The pandemic scrambled day-to-day life for everyone and brought new challenges to academic and clinical settings. It is hard to imagine anything of that magnitude during a normal year. We chose to use the pandemic as a reason for needing Red Team approaches for several of the cases because it is a complex problem with myriad consequences.

However, Red Teaming doesn't require once-in-a-lifetime problems for it to be effective. Rather, it can and should be used whenever multiple perspectives are needed to solve problems, plan or review a project, answer a question, or analyze an issue.

It is helpful to read Chaps. 1, 2, 3, 4, and 5 before moving on to the cases; however, the cases can be read in any order. Although we have written cases that occur in clinical settings and academic settings, the Red Teaming that takes place can be applied in any setting.

Contents

Part I

Why Red Team?

Nursing Leadership in a Segmented Discipline

Why Nursing Leaders Need a New Way to Lead

Nursing has had a long tradition of great leaders. From Florence Nightingale to the leaders of today, the profession has matured and developed because of great leaders who are open to new ideas and challenges. In the 1930s, Effie J. Taylor presented a paper to the National League for Nursing [4] in which she mentioned the need to better prepare nurses for administrative positions. She recommended that nursing experience not be the sole prerequisite for obtaining an administrative position, and that it was necessary to provide predetermined and organized courses specific to administrative responsibilities. She did not discount the need for certain personal characteristics or experience and admitted that some people have particular abilities that make them more likely to be good leaders. The same holds true today. However, we still are likely to advance a nurse to a leadership position because they have been with the organization a long time without necessarily considering whether they have any innate ability or have had sufficient formal preparation for the role.

Additionally, a nurse might receive a promotion to a leadership position due to favoritism or possession of a graduate degree. The profession has developed a general flavor of elitism over the years. Those recruited to be among the elite may not necessarily be the best leaders. They tend to be recognized among the elite by virtue of their education, prestigious position, or their network of colleagues. This author (LNB) recalls working at a very prestigious "top ten" school of nursing (SON) whose dean was an excellent researcher but a terrible leader. Despite numerous faculty letters to the president of the university complaining about her leadership style, she was reappointed because her research brought in generous federal funding. Deans and chairs of nursing, especially, are difficult to find and recruit. Those who are well aware of the responsibilities of these leadership positions may be reluctant to assume them. So others who may not be aware or adequately prepared may be hired into these roles. Also, researchers and others interested in increased recognition within and outside the profession may desire to become chairs or deans but may not necessarily be suited to the role.

© The Author(s), under exclusive license to Springer Nature Switzerland AG 2021
L. Neal-Boylan, S. Rotkoff, *Innovative Decision Making in Healthcare*,
https://doi.org/10.1007/978-3-030-72648-5_1

The bedside nurse rarely has the opportunity for recognition beyond their employing organization. The elite reward the elite or "wanna be" elite. Rarely, if ever, is the nurse who has worked hard to provide quality care to patients but is not a researcher, educator, or in receipt of large amounts of federal funding to receive national recognition. Consequently, those who are elevated to leadership positions and have the most influence over large-scale changes within the organization or profession are often those least in touch with what bedside nurses or nurses on the ground experience or need.

Worse, the leaders at the top of the professional ladder rarely include the voices of those at the bedside or junior academics whether or not they have the opportunity to hear those voices. As nursing sought "a seat at the table" and positions on boards, the profession has become more like a business with a built-in hierarchy that is unnecessary and probably unintended. This is not to say that nurses should not have a seat at the table to serve on boards because the voice of the nursing profession must be heard in discussions that relate to healthcare. However, as the profession has evolved, two separate but equal tiers of nurses have emerged [2]. Associated with each tier are subgroups that are often excluded from high-level discussions that impact the profession.

A House Divided (Box 1.1)

One tier includes the deans and researchers in the "top ten" schools of nursing across the country. In this author's (LNB) experience, merely including the name of one of these SONs on a grant application research proposal or manuscript can almost guarantee success or a higher score regardless of its quality or applicability to practice. In the meantime, other solid applications, proposals, and manuscripts tend to get more scrutiny under review and lower scores. This is especially true for lesser known SONs and departments of nursing, one of the subgroups associated with the first tier. Another group associated with the first tier comprises SONs that are fairly well known and have fairly good grant funding and research proposal and publication acceptance rates. Research nurses who work in prestigious hospitals or academic health centers are another related group.

Box 1.1 Two Tiers in Nursing

Tier 1	Tier 2
Work in higher education	Work at the bedside
Researchers in prestigious institutions	Work in non-clinical settings (not in Tier 1)
Work in academic health center	Work clinically outside the hospital
Attend research conferences	Have a hard time affording attendance at conferences
Read research journals	Read clinically focused journals
Have graduate degrees	Primarily have undergraduate degrees, but some have graduate degrees

The second tier consists of nurses who practice in other settings. Associated with the second tier are groups that include nurses who work full time at the bedside, nurses who work in clinical settings outside the hospital, and nurses who work in non-clinical settings. "Clinical setting" is frequently defined differently depending on who is using the phrase. It can mean anything from direct hands on patient care to case management or advice.

The nursing profession has a tradition of "shooting itself in the foot" by excluding many voices from significant conversations. We often have a hard time making a decision and when we do, we have a hard time making it stick. Take for example, the continued differences in entry-level education and the multitude of nursing education programs that abound. We started out with diploma programs that were excellent in their way because students gained a lot of valuable clinical experience. Speak to a nurse who graduated from a diploma program and it is likely she is an expert clinician even decades after graduation. We then moved on to a few baccalaureate degree (BSN) opportunities and myriad associate degree (ADN) programs. The BSN programs gradually surpassed the ADN programs but many remain. Eventually, the BSN programs winnowed out many hours of clinical practice in lieu of increased emphasis on theory. The focus on theory was vitally important since nurses were becoming scientists and needed to understand the "why" as well as the "how" of nursing practice. However, instead of adding time to the degree such as has been done with the entry-level program in physical therapy, making the entry-level degree a doctor of physical therapy, we limited clinical practice and encouraged students to go on to graduate degrees.

Master's degree programs inadvertently encouraged movement away from bedside nursing; however, this author, over more than 20 years in nursing education, personally heard many faculty tell students to get master's degrees specifically to move away from bedside nursing. We invented direct entry master's programs whereby a student could go directly through to a master's in nursing in 3 years. We now have direct entry doctor in nursing practice and PhD in nursing programs. Consistently reducing student clinical practice and maintaining a multitude of entry-level programs has not only confused the public and our healthcare colleagues, but has contradicted our constant rhetoric that we are a profession on par with physicians and attorneys.

Our nursing organizations have cited rationale for maintaining all these programs and shortening basic nursing education; however, to what extent have these decisions been made with multilevel input from nurses across tiers and associated groups? Admittedly, it is challenging to include the voices across all levels of nursing for several reasons unrelated to lack of motivation. Some nursing organizations have tried hard to include nurses from both tiers in important conversations. Nurses are frequently too busy or overworked to participate in surveys or questionnaires sent out by professional organizations; the cost of attending conferences is frequently exorbitant and unaffordable for many nurses, and some nurses just want to do their work and not be involved. However, there is no doubt that the few are making decisions for the many.

Nursing organizations have made little effort to make conferences affordable and accessible, thereby automatically excluding nurses who cannot afford to attend or work for organizations that cannot afford to cover their expenses. The recent COVID pandemic moved many conferences online, which may be a good model for the future because in several instances, these conferences were free or of low cost. Nurses did not have to pay for transportation, childcare, or hotels in addition to a hefty registration fee and meals. There is no substitute for in-person networking, but the advantage was the likelihood of increased inclusion. We typically use the word "inclusion" with regard to race, ethnicity, and gender identity, but in this case, we should also add position, rank, experience, and education.

In addition, while we may not want to admit it, varying levels of nursing education and the increasing number of quick entry, quick exit programs has resulted in nursing graduates who are not necessarily well educated. We have sometimes lowered standards to admit students, nurtured them to pass [3] and condensed their programs to the extent that they may not be as well prepared as we would like to think, in nursing, in science, or in general education. Consequently, while theoretically any registered nurse should be able to gain knowledge from any nursing conference, many conferences are simply too high level for many nurses.

Similarly, our nursing journals are evidence of the chasm between the first and second tiers. We have research journals that frequently require a PhD to comprehend. While it is necessary for us to publish our research, it has limited value if nurses from the second tier cannot understand and apply it. Conversely, first-tier nurses are unlikely to read clinical journals unless they maintain a clinical practice in addition to their full-time work. Frequently, the result is that second-tier nurses do not access research findings that might enhance the quality of their practice and first-tier nurses are unaware of what is actually happening in clinical practice and how to direct their research to improve it or the worklife of nurses.

This segmentation between the first and second tiers coupled with the hierarchies that exist within each subgroup precludes productive and inclusive conversation. There are two hierarchies within the academic setting: the administrative hierarchy and the rank hierarchy. The first hierarchy is characterized by a combination of the administrative levels that may include track coordinator, program director, assistant dean, associate dean, and dean or department chair. In addition, there are committees that must approve basic actions, such as new course proposals, that must also acquire university approval.

The second hierarchy is inherent in the promotion and tenure system. "Clinical" or "adjunct" faculty, often one and the same, may or may not sit on SON committees or vote on SON decisions. Yet, they frequently are the most current in the reality of clinical practice. Junior faculty, hoping to get tenure and promotion, are reluctant to publicly disagree with senior faculty who have a lot of influence over promotion and tenure decisions. Junior faculty who are hired because they are inclined to innovative thinking and modern ideas are often prevented from voicing them because senior faculty like the way things are done, do not want to exert the energy required by change or are skeptical of the need for change.

Tenure track faculty, whether assistant or associate professors, walk a fine line because their status is viewed as "eventually to be tenured." However, they too fear retribution when the time comes for promotion and tenure. This is not to mention the secretaries and administrative support staff in SONs and clinical settings who frequently have no voice at all.

In some universities, an SON dean is outranked by a college dean who is not a nurse or the chair of a nursing department who is a nurse is outranked by a dean who is not a nurse. This automatically sets the stage for a potentially adversarial relationship because the nurse chair or dean believes they know what is best for nursing and nursing education and the non-nurse superior thinks nursing education has too many rules and regulations and that these can easily be circumvented or ignored.

Clinical settings also have inherent hierarchies. Leaders promoted from within who have little to no experience or education in leadership or management may be promoted due to their longevity within the organization or their clinical expertise. Others may be hired into leadership positions because they have a graduate degree in leadership or administration but may have little experience in the clinical area they have been asked to manage. I recall interviewing a candidate for a nursing leadership position in an outpatient clinic. The candidate had 1 year of nursing school, entered a master's in nursing program and graduated after 1 year with a master's in nursing with a focus on program outcomes. The nurse had taken courses in leadership theory, quality improvement, and outcomes assessment and had 6 weeks of school clinical experience in a hospital, but had never worked as a nurse. Nonetheless, she had applied for a position managing nursing staff and the non-nurses within the organization supported her candidacy. Our ongoing abbreviation of nursing programs has not served to advance the profession but has moved people with little to no knowledge or experience in nursing into positions that give them significant responsibility for personnel and clinical decisions.

Good Leaders and Not So Good Leaders

Leaders in business and educational organizations often claim that either someone is a good leader or not and their skills can be transferred to any setting. They may think a good leader does not necessarily need to have expertise in whatever is being produced. This may be true in business but not in nursing education or clinical nursing. Nursing is a service profession and requires specific knowledge and skills. A non-nurse leader is likely to misunderstand the need for our stringent requirements. General Dwight D. Eisenhower stated: "The essence of leadership is to get others to do something because they think you want it done and because they know it is worth while doing...." (Remarks at the Republican Campaign Picnic at the President's Gettysburg Farm, 9/12/56; https://www.eisenhowerlibrary.gov/eisenhowers/ quotes). It is much harder for a non-nurse to help nurses understand how what they are being asked to do is worthwhile doing.

The Danger of Groupthink

There are barriers in both academic and non-academic settings to diverging from groupthink or freedom to speak one's mind without potentially risking one's career. Groupthink refers to a phenomenon in which the group makes a decision that discourages innovation or creativity (https://www.google.com/search?client=firefox-b-1-d&q=groupthink+definition). An amusing example of groupthink comes from the military. During the Spanish American War, the cavalry, consisting of soldiers and their trained cavalry horses, were on a ship. The soldiers needed to get the horses to the shore nearby and since horses are good swimmers, they let the horses off the ship. To their dismay, the lead horse headed for the ocean rather than the shore and all the other horses followed him. The soldiers were in a tizzy about what to do. Several of them rode one of the horses out to the lead horse to try to get him to turn around. Others swam out to the horses and tried to lead them in the opposite direction. All, to no avail. Finally, someone thought to play the bugle call for retreat and the lead horse turned around and led all the horses safely to shore.

While horses are known to be smart animals, they followed the leader even if doing so was clearly dangerous and did not make any sense. We are not much better when we trust, respect, or fear our leaders. We may know a better way but think we are too junior in rank or too inexperienced to voice an opinion. Good leaders encourage multiple perspectives even when they are contrary to their own opinions. They value input and are aware the best decision is one that has had input from everyone who has a stake in the success of the decision. In recent years, the nursing literature has used buzzwords, such as transformational leadership and transparent leadership. However, even good leaders cannot always be transformational or transparent. What they can be, however, is inclusive. Red Teaming, when used correctly ensures that all stakeholders are included and the outcome is the best decision that could be made at the time.

Learning to Lead

Today, nursing students begin to learn about leadership in baccalaureate programs and learn advanced methods and models in their masters and doctoral programs. However, those in ADN programs learn leadership later, on the job. Supervisors, managers, and deans model their leadership techniques, for better or worse, during their interactions with their staff, faculty, students, and colleagues. There are myriad books and resources that describe models of leadership and how one becomes a great leader. Some of the best have been written by nurses. Dr. Angela Barron McBride wrote in *The Growth and Development of Nurse Leaders*: "so much is expected of leaders these days that you have to be a brave soul to admit to being one" [1, p. XVI]. She wrote that leaders are often described as heroes and expected to be perfect and not make any mistakes which is clearly impossible and discourages many would-be leaders.

Leadership is a challenge, without question and that is why many nurses seek leadership opportunities. They believe they are ready for a new challenge. Many take on a leadership role without knowing or understanding exactly what will be expected and that the nurse must metamorphosize into someone who is expected to be able to solve everyone's problems while also making everyone happy. Only those who have experienced a leadership role truly understand that you can never please everyone and it is unrealistic to try. To cope with the stress of leadership, the nurse must understand that previous relationships will change and the familiarity and closeness the nurse cherished will frequently dissipate as subordinates begin to recognize the nurse in a different role.

The smart nurse leader recognizes that providing everyone with an opportunity to voice their concerns goes a long way toward helping others feel they have been heard. Some leaders claim they are eliciting and listening to the voices of all employees, but rarely is this true. Gathering faculty, for example, in a room and asking if there are any questions, is not actively hearing everyone's voices. Failing to include administrative assistants and others who implement leadership decisions also fails to capture everyone's voice. Furthermore, listening to the voices but not actually considering them in the final decision is simply paying lip service to good communication and leadership.

Regardless of the abilities of the leader in academic or clinical settings, leaders can only benefit from including the voices of those whom they are expected to lead in discussions and decision-making. However, leaders must first understand their own roles and what it means to be a leader. Deference to the boss and the perks that may be associated with the job only go so far and are quickly replaced with the burden of 24 hour responsibility for decisions ranging from how much paper to order to hiring, firing, and cancelling programs and initiatives due to insufficient funding.

How Red Teaming Fits

The business and nursing literature is replete with advice about how to lead. Many of the methods described in the literature are tried and true. However, nursing leaders need a new way to think and act. It is necessary to recognize that even the flattest organizations have an embedded hierarchy. Without new tools and methods, hierarchy will lead to some level of self-censorship by those in junior positions or lack of responsiveness by those in more senior positions. Red Teaming is a strategy borrowed from the military and subsequently adopted by some in the corporate world. It is an innovative approach to decision-making that should help nursing leaders think in an entirely different way. Please see the preface to this book for a detailed account of how Red Teaming developed.

Why should military and corporate models and approaches be applied to nursing and healthcare settings and organizations? The rate of change in our hyperconnected world has reduced the effective half-life of many decisions. As soon as an organization begins to act, everyone in the environment observes the action and reacts in real time, sharing that reaction with others affected. As a consequence, the environment against which the decision was made rapidly changes into something new. This means that while leaders still need to make decisions, they need to do so while keeping an open mind to the likelihood that circumstances will change rapidly once they act. The military adopted Red Teaming methods to address this new reality. Red Teaming strives to foster divergent conversations before deciding what actions to take. This builds agility into the decision-making process as it allows leaders to recognize a wider spectrum of options before acting, this allows them to be more flexible in their thinking as the situation continues to evolve. These tools are designed to encourage innovation, reduce conflict, increase collaboration, and make the best use of diverse perspectives.

Chapters 3 and 4 describe Red Team tools and methods, and the chapters that follow present cases using Red Team tools. Before we present these cases, it is important to lay some groundwork. First, the cases are intended to illustrate application, but the issues and problems presented in the cases are not simple ones. Red Team methods are offered as innovative alternatives to what we currently do and might not always be effective. However, it is important to remember that the issues and problems have been somewhat simplified to fit within the case analysis. These situations are complex, and each one requires in-depth thought and planning. That said, Red Team methods and tools are applicable to work through these complex issues. There is simply not enough room in this book to address every possible nuance or variable that might arise when working with individuals with varying capabilities and personalities. Every good leader knows there is no one-size-fits-all approach to managing conflict or resolving problems. However, *Red Team tools enable the leader to reach the best solution.*

Some of the cases take place in academic settings, others in clinical settings; however, the Red Team methods chosen to work through each case can be applied to either setting. Many of the conflicts encountered by nurse leaders revolve around personnel conflicts, future planning, and budget cuts and restrictions. We have endeavored to apply Red Team tools to these critical issues.

While Red Team tools are applicable to both clinical and academic settings, there are some considerations when using the tools. The rest of this chapter focuses on these specific considerations.

Clinical Settings

Clinical settings, regardless whether in outpatient or inpatient settings consist of nurses and other staff with varying educational backgrounds. Registered nurses (RN) may have a diploma, bachelor's degree, master's degree, or doctorate (DNP or PhD). Licensed practical nurses (LPN), medical assistants, and certified nurse's aides (CNA) may not have any college education. Unit secretaries are likely to have scant medical expertise. In addition, healthcare has become increasingly interprofessional, so a clinical leader might employ Red Team methods with interdisciplinary groups whose educational backgrounds vary significantly. Clinical experiences will also vary in length and type.

It is important that clinical leaders be aware of and sensitive to these distinctions. Red Team methods ensure everyone has a voice so leaders must ensure that hierarchies created by education, experience, or position do not interfere with application of Red Team tools.

In addition, nurses working in clinical settings have increased exposure to death and disease. Along with differences in education, experience, and position, exposure to death and disease might compel some nurses to think they have a greater stake in the solution than other nurses or staff. Also, exposure to disease might cause attrition of stakeholders in important Red Team meetings because the nurses themselves become ill and cannot go to work.

Some clinical settings operate on multiple shifts and with varying work hours. Gathering stakeholders to address an issue or problem can be challenging. Patient care is the primary purpose of a clinical setting, so sufficient staffing is necessary at all times. Emergencies, inservice education, Joint Commission, and Magnet reviews can all interfere with attempts to gather the relevant stakeholders on multiple occasions.

While leaders must be sensitive to these interferences, a problem to which Red Team tools are being applied is likely to be of some significance. There must be time dedicated to using the tools appropriately.

Academic Settings

While in academic settings, faculty tend to have a minimum of a master's degree if not a doctorate, they vary in levels of experience in both nursing and academe. If staff are included in meetings that use Red Team tools, then leaders must consider the potentially significant difference between faculty and staff educational backgrounds.

Although faculty are not exposed to death and disease in the same way as clinical nurses, faculty perceive differences in their entitlement and privilege based on rank, tenure status, and whether or not they are considered "clinical" or "research" faculty. Research faculty who bring grant funding to the school of nursing might perceive that their voices should count for more than those of other faculty. Once again, leaders must be careful to use Red Team methods to ensure that all pertinent voices are heard and given equal opportunity to speak. This is why Red Team methods are so important to academic environments. They can help leaders overcome the natural barriers presented by academic hierarchies.

SONs vary with regard to how much or how often adjuncts or part-time faculty are included in decision-making processes. When the topic of discussion is relevant to their work with students, adjuncts should be permitted to have an equal voice if not an equal vote. Red Team methods and tools are perfect for this.

Another point of consideration in academic settings is that beyond rank, experience and whether or not faculty are primarily focused on research, teaching, or clinical practice, faculty frequently have additional roles, such as department chair, program director, assistant, or associate dean. Faculty members might be lab coordinators or course coordinators. These positions may identify a faculty member as a stakeholder in a particular situation requiring Red Team intervention; however, the position itself should not denote more influence in resolving the problem or issue than any other stakeholder.

Consider this book a "how-to" book regarding use of an innovative method (Red Teaming) to reach the best decision. At first, it may seem cumbersome to use these tools but, as in most things worth doing, they will become second nature. It is ideal if your school or clinical setting can afford to hire a Red Team consultant; however, you can learn to apply the tools and refine them using trial and error.

Red Teaming cannot "unsegment" nursing. That is not its purpose. Regardless of whether you apply Red Team tools to a clinical or academic setting, ultimately, the person in charge has the final say. Red Teaming does not remove that power. The ultimate authority invested in the leader remains, but Red Teaming makes the leader's job easier by arriving at the best solution and being truly transparent and inclusive. The best idea wins.

Nursing considers innovation important. This is true with regard to our curricula, our research, and our clinical practice. We are innovators by nature and we are great at adapting to new ways of doing things once we are convinced they are worth our time and effort. Try these tools and begin to think of nursing leadership in a different way.

References

1. McBride AB. The growth and development of nurse leaders. New York: Springer; 2011.
2. Neal-Boylan L. The nurse's reality shift: using our history to transform our future. Indianapolis: Sigma Theta Tau Publishing; 2014.
3. Neal-Boylan L, Miller M, Lussier-Duynstee P. Failing to fail when disability is a factor. Nurse Educ. 2020; https://doi.org/10.1097/NNE.0000000000000965.
4. Taylor EJ. Address of President Effie J. Taylor. Proceedings of the fortieth annual convention of the NLNE, 1934, Washington, D.C. Of what is the nature of nursing? NLN Publ. Washington, DC: National League for Nursing. 1993;(14-2514):277–82.

Why Red Teaming Is a Better Way

2

As we set the stage for discussing Red Team approaches in detail and applying them to several cases, it is important to discuss why Red Team approaches are preferable to other methods when considering the future of organizations. Modern planning and decision-making must cope with the following four dichotomies on a regular basis.

First, is the age-old struggle between near term planning, when the environment looks similar to that during which the plan is being formed and long-term planning, when the world may be very different from today. While this challenge is not new, the greatly increased rate of change in the environment makes this problem unlike that of the past.

Second, while the rate of change in our surrounding world has increased dramatically, the rate of change in human behavior remains slow. Humans are pack animals, and it is often difficult to stimulate creative thought and think about alternative futures while part of the pack; groupthink takes over. "Groupthink is a psychological drive for consensus at any cost that suppresses dissent and appraisal of alternatives in cohesive decision making groups" [2, p. 8].

As described by Irving Janis in his seminal work *Groupthink* [3], the following are the eight characteristics common in this phenomenon:

- *Illusions of invulnerability*: The belief that the group cannot fail.
- *Morality*: The belief that the group's motives are inherently good and correct.
- *Rationalizing*: The tendency to "explain away" contradictory information or data.
- *Stereotyping*: The tendency to portray others who are opposed to the group as evil or stupid.
- *Self-censorship*: The tendency of group members to keep their doubts to themselves.
- *Illusions of unanimity*: The belief that silence is the same as agreement.
- *Mindguards*: The emergence of self-appointed thought police who actively shield the group from information that might challenge its assumptions.
- *Conformity*: The tendency to view dissent as disloyalty.

© The Author(s), under exclusive license to Springer Nature Switzerland AG 2021
L. Neal-Boylan, S. Rotkoff, *Innovative Decision Making in Healthcare*,
https://doi.org/10.1007/978-3-030-72648-5_2

If the boss says, "I think we ought to consider X," most subordinates will immediately think of how best to implement X without even taking a moment to consider whether X is a good idea. Even the most benevolent bosses influence employees in this way, sometimes without saying a word. Frequently, body language or facial expressions can clue us in to what our seniors want. These effects are often subconscious, but nonetheless influence our actions. This kind of behavior and other manifestations of groupthink are the death of creative thinking required to prosper in the coming future.

Third, is that we tend to promote people who are extremely good at tactical thinking into positions that require strategic thinking. This was famously captured in the "Peter Principal." The Peter Principle refers to a book by the same name published by Laurence J. Peter. It is defined as the principle that members of a hierarchical organization are promoted until they reach the level at which they are no longer competent [6].

A key ingredient in the military method for growing leaders is a conscious management of individuals' exposure to different types of leadership challenges. The skills required to run a single unit and those required to run a hospital are not the same. The military has coped with this challenge for millennia in growing novice Lieutenants into General officers over time. It is very difficult in the military to ascend to the highest ranks without having a broad base of experience. It is why we call senior officers Generals; they are generalists by design and have served in different environments. They have served as both staff and senior executives; they understand administration, logistics, and operations.

Despite hundreds of years of experience and a concerted effort to avoid promoting people beyond their capacity, the Army still sometimes gets it wrong. This happens for a variety of reasons. Leaders are evaluated by their seniors. Often a leader looks great to the boss but is despised by their subordinates. At times, this disconnect is not revealed until the leader has achieved more authority than they should. Leaders being human, sometimes change. As they get older, the energy and innovation they displayed as a junior leader may fade. Some leaders are great at either surrounding themselves with others who are smarter than they are, or taking credit for their subordinates' work. When they are put in a situation where they must stand on their own merits, they are revealed to be less than they seemed. This is just as true in nursing.

Finally, we all suffer from "sunk cost bias." Once we spend a lot of time and energy thinking about how to build a plan, we are loath to let go of that plan, even if the environment has changed significantly. The challenge is building a detailed plan while remaining agile in execution as the environment continues to evolve. As General of the Army Dwight Eisenhower once said "plans are worthless, but planning is everything" [1] (https://quoteinvestigator.com/2017/11/18/planning/#note-17261-5). Before continuing, take a moment to reflect on your own experience in nursing or healthcare. Have you ever experienced any of the four dichotomies described above and listed below?

> **Box 2.1 Goals of Building Alternatives**
> 1. Diverge thinking before converging on a course of action.
> 2. Ensure selection of the best idea versus the one with the most powerful advocate.
> 3. Enable the planning team to remain agile during implementation.

1. A focus on near-term planning at the exclusion of long-term consequences.
2. Groupthink stifling the consideration of a wide range of options and narrowly focusing on what the boss wants.
3. Planning led by leaders who try and apply inappropriate or outdated personal experience to a problem they do not fully understand.
4. An unwillingness to change the plan after the circumstances around the problem have changed in a way the plan did not anticipate.

Red Teaming utilizes a series of tools and methods designed to generate alternative perspectives around how to solve a problem or develop a plan. The goals of building alternatives is threefold (Box 2.1): First, to diverge in our thinking before we converge on a course of action; second, to ensure we select the best idea instead of the idea with the most powerful advocate; and third, to enable the planning team to remain agile during execution if the future unfolds differently than expected.

Divergence Before Convergence

Myriad studies [4, 5, 7] of human decision-making attest to the reality that we do not, as a rule, deliberately weigh options and select the best course of action. Some of us do this occasionally when making a large purchase like a home or a car, but even those of us who build lists comparing options side by side are often influenced by emotional or irrational factors while making the decision. While emotional considerations in decision-making are frequent, we do not often recognize the emotional component of our decision-making. It is a fairly common experience for someone to have a long list of desired attributes for their house purchase that they simply ignore, because the sunroom reminds them of the house they lived in as a kid.

More insidious than emotion is when we think our approach is completely rational, when in reality it is simply the first approach we think of that might work. This author (SR) experienced an example of this when buying a house after retiring from the Army. When first retiring, it was necessary to move to Washington DC, while my wife cleared out of our military housing. I had a list of things the new house needed to have. The first was that the house had to meet certain commuter criteria in terms of time required to make it to my new job each day. The second was that it had to have room for all of our household goods. Third, it had to be within a certain price range, and finally it had to be in a nice neighborhood with convenient shopping nearby. A bonus was if it had a homeowners' club with a gym and pool. On the second day of looking for new homes, I came upon a house that met all five criteria (to include the homeowners' club) and put in an offer. Once the criteria I had identified were met, I essentially stopped looking at any other possible homes. My focus on the five criteria resulted in me being oblivious to the hideous color scheme and the fact that the house was four stories high with the master bedroom at the top, and the laundry at the bottom. There is a name for premature seizing on a solution. It is called "satificing."

Gary Klein [5] in, *Sources of Power: How people make decisions* (after years of research in the field following fire fighters as they made decisions), proposes that most of us "satifice." Satifysing is the act of adopting the very first solution to a problem that seems to fit. This is often not the optimum solution. It is simply the first one we think of that will work. Often we are drawn to these options because they are familiar; it is what we have done in the past when faced with a similar problem. As long as the problem we confront is routine, this approach is practical and will work. When we face a new problem that is substantially different from things we have experienced in the past, that is a challenge. In these cases, unless we use some vehicle to force ourselves to thoroughly think through the problem and recognize the difference, we will gravitate to a solution that has worked in the past and apply it to a problem set for which it is ill suited. (In the case of buying the house, part of the reason I "satificed" is that I had never encountered a condo, and while I had bought houses before, they were all one or two stories, so the architectural layout had never been a significant consideration).

Red Team approaches address this problem by forcing everyone to think quietly about the nature of the problem and then individually develop their solutions, driving the group to a divergent approach. It is only after the group has created a broad and imaginative collection of approaches to the issue through divergence that tools are then used to converge from a wide variety of solutions to the family of best solutions. This approach ensures that *satisficing* does not occur. Note, this approach is not recommended when fighting a fire. When in the middle of an emergency situation, best practices and drills are always the best approach. However, many problems are not urgent; those that require planning and thought are the most appropriate for Red Teaming. If my wife had been with me when I bought the house, the kind of divergent thought required to identify the poor color scheme and the multiple stories would have occurred as a consequence of our dialogue.

Chapter 3 introduces a series of tools designed to assist planners to consider alternative perspectives and increase divergence of thought. This class of tools is called "Changing the Frame of Reference."

Ensuring the Best Idea Wins

As pack animals, humans prefer to be with other humans, and we are highly socialized to identify the pecking order inside of any group. Most of us can remember trying to determine who had the power in the group, who were the "cool kids" and who the outsiders were, who was successful, and who was less so. Watch any group of kids on the playground and you will see an "alpha" kid who decides what everyone will play and other kids who try to be close with the alpha, while some will operate outside the group. It is the very nature of our human condition. This affects our decision-making and planning as even the most benevolent bosses can influence their subordinates without saying a word. A raised eyebrow or crossing arms or legs are among signals to the group regarding what the boss wants. When this happens, the group reflects back to the boss the idea the boss wanted to begin with. Even when pressed for time, if the boss provides guidance, then leaves the room and allows their subordinates to discuss the issue in their absence, the result will almost always be a more open discussion and a better plan.

Some ideas win simply because their advocate is the best speaker and can argue rings around someone who may have a stronger plan but weaker rhetoric. Another tactic used in planning groups is to simply have more stamina than your opponents. Many advocates have given up their support of an idea or opposition to a different idea simply because they were tired of the argument and wanted to go home. Red Team tools preclude this from happening. One of the Red Team mantras is "no silver backed gorillas in the room!" A "silver backed gorilla" in the wild is that dominant male who beats his chest, bares his teeth, and intimidates the troop to do what he wants.

But what if the boss' idea, or the smooth talker's idea, or the persistent advocate's idea is not the best? What if that same idea, were it proffered by someone else, would not gain widespread endorsement? How does the group ensure the BEST ideas win, not the idea with the most powerful or loudest advocate?

Chapter 3 introduces several tools and methods specifically designed to address this problem. This class of tools is called "Liberating Structures." These are structured methods for liberating conversations from the constraints of hierarchy and groupthink.

Remaining Agile in Execution

No matter how much we plan, the future always seems to have a mind of its own. All of the following are common items which can quickly and without much warning change the trajectory of the future into one for which we did not plan:

- A new technology emerges that makes our approach, built around a current technology, outdated.
- A key person in our plan implementation structure departs for unforeseen reasons.
- An external action occurs over which we have no control (e.g., legal or policy changes that we cannot affect, unexpected impacts on funding, data breaches, and a pandemic).
- We discover one of the assumptions upon which we built our plan is no longer true.
- A competitor working independently can offer a solution that makes our plan moot.

All of these things have happened to large and well-established businesses, many of which continued to execute their plan as if nothing unusual had happened to derail that plan. These businesses went the way of Blockbuster, Polaroid, and Blackberry. Chapter 4 introduces a set of tools specifically designed to envision alternative futures. This class of tools is called "Envisioning Alternative Futures."

Solving the Right Problem

It is important to be working on the right problem to be solved. Too often in both nursing academe and in clinical settings, people become focused on the wrong problem. Nurses may think the problem is that no one is using the appropriate equipment, but the actual problem may be related to communication and the interactions of the people involved in ordering the equipment.

Another example might involve diabetic patients. Most of the patients are diabetic in the community clinic in which this author works (LNB). We teach patients to make lifestyle changes that will lower blood sugar and prevent complications of the disease. We also treat patients with medications and teach them to monitor their blood sugar using a blood glucose monitor. Our protocol is to have patients' follow-up in the clinic every 3–4 months; however, many of our patients do not return to the clinic for longer periods. We typically interpret this as lack of willingness to take the time to follow-up, non-adherence to the prescribed regimen, and/or inability to pay for a follow-up visit despite the discounted cost. However, another cause could be and has frequently been that patients are following their regimen, have made lifestyle changes, and are seeing improved results when they check their blood sugar levels at home. They do not think they need to follow-up or continue to take their medications because they are doing better. Chapter 4 introduces tools specifically aimed at *root cause analysis* and understanding the problem to be solved.

Conclusion

The application of the tools described in the next two chapters will ensure better decisions are made, decision-makers acknowledge that the outcomes of those decisions are not preordained, and the organization remains flexible in an era of rapidly changing events. Having described the "why" of Red Teaming, the next two chapters (Chaps. 3 and 4) will describe each of the tools and how they are used. Many of these tools are so simple you can begin applying them immediately, others build upon the simplest tools and will require some practice. Every tool will be illustrated in application. These applications are embedded in a series of case studies. All of the case studies take place either in a school of nursing or a clinical setting. We highly recommend you read Chaps. 3 and 4 before the case studies as the cases will be much easier to follow if you are familiar with the tools. As you read the rest of this book, we urge you to think of your own applications – both to issues you have confronted in the past and those you confront today. Ask yourself if a specific tool might have led to a better conversation, more divergent thought, more creative idea generation, or more agile execution during unfolding of an unanticipated future.

References

1. Blair W. President draws planning moral: recalls army days to show value of preparedness in time of crisis. New York Times. November 29, 1957.
2. Janis I. Victims of groupthink: psychological study of foreign policy decisions and fiascos. Boston: Houghton-Mifflin; 1972.
3. Janis I. Groupthink. Boston: Wadsworth; 1982.
4. Kahneman D. Thinking fast and thinking slow. New York: Farrar, Straus & Giroux; 2011.
5. Klein GA. Sources of power: how people make decisions. Cambridge, MA: MIT Press; 1999. ISBN 0-262-61146-5.
6. Peter LJ, Hull R. The Peter principle. New York: Harper Collins Publishers; 2009.
7. Senge P. The fifth discipline: the art & practice of the learning organization. New York: Random House; 1990.

The Red Team Toolbox: Improving the Conversation and Changing the Frame of Reference

3

Red Team methods are powerful because you can use them all the time, irrespective of whether the group is actually conducting a planning exercise. Better conversations that include more people result in improved morale and a sense of ownership by all members of the organization. *Red Team tools challenge people to embrace divergence before convergence, mitigate groupthink, and ensure the best idea wins.* The issues that face decision-making people or groups are fundamentally consequences of normal human behavior. However, analyzing or resolving them cannot be done without intentional methods or approaches. To cultivate new ideas and increase inclusion, it is necessary to use methods designed to change the dynamics of conversations (Fig. 3.1).

Liberating Structures

The meta concept around these tools is called *liberating structures* (LS) because the goal is to liberate the conversation through use of a structured methodology. LS does not include informal gatherings and brainstorming that many people consider the means to encourage divergent thought.

In this book, we focus on two specific types of liberating structures: (1) those designed to enable divergent thought and creative approaches to problem solving and (2) those designed to help the group converge on the best idea by leveraging the wisdom of the entire group (Box 3.1). These are by no means the only liberating structures. Any method designed to get people to tell the hard truth about a problem using *think-write-share*, anonymous participation, or some other divergent method, coupled with a means to ensure the best idea wins, may be called a liberating structure. The exact same method can be conducted in both a *liberating structure* style and a non-liberating structure style. When we explain *premortem analysis,* we will illustrate that difference.

© The Author(s), under exclusive license to Springer Nature Switzerland AG 2021
L. Neal-Boylan, S. Rotkoff, *Innovative Decision Making in Healthcare*,
https://doi.org/10.1007/978-3-030-72648-5_3

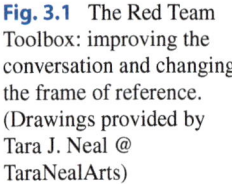

Fig. 3.1 The Red Team Toolbox: improving the conversation and changing the frame of reference. (Drawings provided by Tara J. Neal @ TaraNealArts)

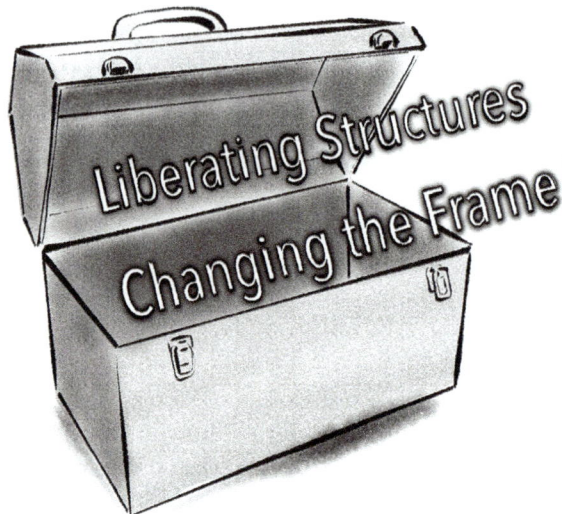

Box 3.1 Liberating Structures to Cultivate Divergence or Convergence
- Think-write-share – divergence.
- 1-2-4-all – divergence.
- Round Robin – divergence.
- A team – B team – divergence.
- 5 will get you 25 – convergence.
- Dot voting – convergence.
- Forced distribution – convergence.
- Best of breed – convergence.

For our purposes, we define divergent thinking as: "Thinking that may follow many lines of thought and tends to generate new and original solutions to problems" (https://www.merriam-webster.com/dictionary). Convergent thinking is defined as "thinking that weighs alternatives within an existing construct to find one best solution" (https://www.merriam-webster.com/dictionary/).

Tools to Cultivate Divergent Thinking

Think-Write-Share (T-W-S)

This tool is designed to slow down thinking to allow reflection and increased reasoning. It also prevents grandstanding, thinking out loud, unconsidered commentary, and group members from seizing the rhetorical initiative and driving the conversation in their desired direction. It is as simple as it sounds.

1. *Think*: Spend some time mulling over the issue or question. Take mental excursions around different possibilities. Try to think for at least 5 minutes. Forcing yourself to think for an extended period will open your mind to ideas you might preemptively dismiss.
2. *Write*: Write your thoughts down. This does not have to be an extensive explanation. Do not self-censor. The act of writing for most people helps refine their ideas
3. *Share in small groups*: If time allows, the best way to share ideas is to break the larger group into groups of two. Discussions of ideas among two people have a special quality. Neither person can sit out the discussion. Even the most introverted or least confident will speak up in a group of two. Building up from two to larger groups will allow those uncomfortable in the larger groups to be represented by those they spoke with in the smaller group. This way everyone is heard at least once. When time does not allow groups of two, try to hold initial discussions in as small a group as possible.

1-2-4-All

This method is a specific application of T-W-S in small groups. After conducting T-W-S in groups of two, aggregate groups of two into groups of four, keeping paired teams together. After the teams have worked to develop solutions to the question posed, have each team select a spokesperson. Rotate spokespeople among the teams, so that the spokesperson briefs another team as to what his/ her team developed and then fields questions or notes suggestions using *Yes, and...* to improve the plan. After rotation, spokespeople return to their original group to refine the original solution. This culminates with each group sharing their ideas with the entire group in plenary. This method is best used with groups of 12 or more.

Round Robin

Frequently during brainstorming, a few voices will dominate. Round Robin is designed to combat that tendency. After everyone has individually addressed the question using the *T-W-S* methodology, the facilitator will ask for input by going around the room allowing each person to only share one idea they developed. If a person who has not spoken, hears one of their ideas proffered by another member of the group, they cross that idea off their own list. *Everyone speaks once before anyone speaks twice*. This is continued until every idea has been captured. The result is a divergent list of approaches developed independently and representing everyone. *Round Robin* is frequently followed by *dot voting* as a means to converge on the best idea of those developed by the group.

A Team B Team

This tool was first used by an aerospace company. The company was bidding for a large government contract to build a next-generation fighter airplane. There was a rift among the company engineers as to how to proceed with two camps, each advocating for a very different kind of design to represent the company's offering in their bid to the government. The company decided to break the engineers into two completely separated teams. Each team would build their proposed airplane. Each team would then brief the company board of directors. Both teams were given the same guidelines to inform their presentations. They had to make the best possible case for their aircraft design and make the case against their competitor's approach. They also had to provide the same administrative information, such as, cost and maintenance. The result of this *A team B team approach* was that the board was able to take some ideas from both groups and improve the design to be the most competitive. This company won the bid from the government and their approach has since become a standard, taught in numerous MBA programs.

Weighted Anonymous Feedback (WAF)

WAF tools leverage the power of anonymity to get groups to grade the ideas collected from divergence and converge on those ideas the group thinks are the best ideas. *Dot voting, 5 will get you 25,* and *forced distribution* all provide WAF. This is how to ensure the Best IDEA versus the idea with the Best Advocate wins!

Convergence

5 Will Get You 25

This is a fun way of getting WAF. The object is to both separate the source of the idea from the idea and gather the wisdom of the crowd around the best idea.

Step 1: Craft a question that can be answered with a single recommendation. The question should be critical to solving the problem and one, if voiced aloud, might require people to self-censor instead of telling the truth. See Box 3.2 for examples of some of the questions used with this technique.

> **Box 3.2 Potential Questions to Use with the Tool *5 Will Get You 25***
> - What is the single greatest challenge we face in implementing this new system?
> - What is the single biggest lie we tell ourselves about who we are or what we do?
> - Who/what is the single greatest risk we must confront to make this change?

Note that phrases "single greatest, single biggest or single most" are always part of the question because you want to limit people to one answer instead of a laundry list of responses. This is necessary for the tool to work, but also forces people to prioritize their responses.

Step 2: The facilitator hands out different colored index cards to each member of the team and gives everyone in the entire group pens identical in style and color. The object is always to separate the source of the idea from the idea. If Suzy, for example, is known for using a green pen, we want to ensure she uses the exact same black as everyone else.

Step 3: The facilitator gives the initial set of instructions:

- You may only write on the front side of the card (it helps if the index cards are lined on one side and that side is designated the front).
- You must write legibly as others will have to read what you write.
- If you have very distinctive handwriting that others might identify, please block print instead.
- Keep your response professional; no personal attacks.
- After you have written your answer, please stand up and move to the center of the room taking your card and pen with you.

Step 4: Once everyone is standing, the facilitator begins the process of weighting the anonymous feedback

- Everyone circulates around the room randomly changing cards with everyone they pass until the facilitator says *STOP* (Fig. 3.2).
- Cards are passed with the text side up.
- For the initial exchange, everyone must end the mixing with a different colored card than the one with which they started (they can exchange with a neighbor, if this is not the case when you say "stop"). See Box 3.3 regarding how the facilitator enables step four.

Box 3.3 Instructions for the Facilitator

If you have an even number of people, then you hand out two different colors of cards.

If you have an odd number of participants, then use three different colors of cards. Once everyone has a card that is not their own (different color), instruct them as follows:

Read the card and firmly fix in your head the quality of the idea. Rate a great idea with the number 5; a good idea with the number 4; terrible ideas with the number 1; poor or mediocre ideas with numbers 2 or 3, respectively.

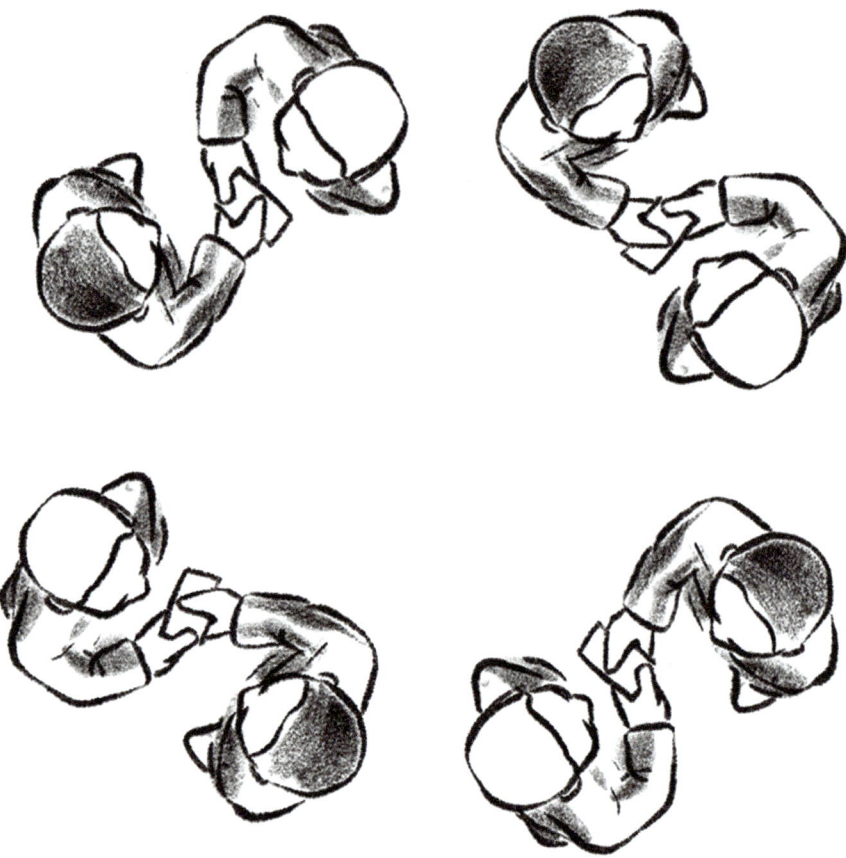

Fig. 3.2 Circulating and passing index cards

Step 5: The rules change a little after the initial mixing is complete:

- Once again, everyone moves around the room and exchanges cards until the facilitator says *STOP*. Participants should hold the card with the idea face up, so they do not see the side of the card with the grade (1–5) given the idea. Unlike the first mixing, the color of the card no longer matters.
- Once the facilitator says *STOP*, everyone must stop and read their card to themselves but *NOT* grade it until directed. Anyone who either receives their own card back *OR* receives a card they previously graded raises their hand and states "I cannot grade this card." They *SHOULD NOT* say "this is my card, I cannot grade it," since the object of this exercise is to truly separate the source of the idea from the idea and ensure separate and independent grading. Those who have cards they cannot grade will exchange with others in the group until everyone publicly confirms that they have a "gradeable" card.
- Once everyone has a "gradeable" card, the facilitator reminds them to evaluate the idea and determine their individual grade of the idea before turning the card over. He then says, "grade your cards," which they do (Fig. 3.3).

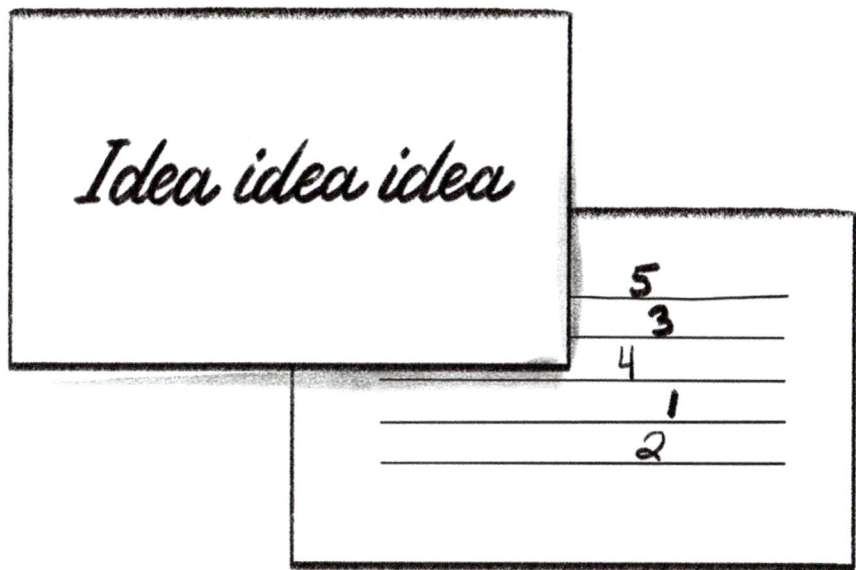

Fig. 3.3 5 will get you 25

Box 3.4 Why Use *5 Will Get You 25* Early in Planning?
- It establishes early on that this is not a typical brainstorming session since the methods are different.
- It establishes the importance of anonymity along with weighted feedback.
- It identifies early, the things about which people in the room are most concerned.

Note: it is very important that the facilitator think through and craft the best thought-provoking, single-answer question in order to get the most value from this method (Box 3.3).

Step 6: Repeat step 5 until the cards have been graded at least by one-third plus 1 of the total group size (in a group of 12, this will result in 5 grades on the back of each card).

Step 7: The facilitator has everyone return to their seats and totals the numbers on the back of each card.

Any idea that averages a grade more than four is an idea the group must confront. This means the wisdom of the group (the original writer along with more than one-third the sample size) considered this idea as real and important. Box 3.4 lists why this tool is frequently used early in the planning process.

Dot Voting

Dot voting is the simplest convergence technique.

Step 1: After using some other LS divergence tool, such as *T-W-S* or *1-2-4-all* to collect a large number of recommendations, the group must collectively combine similar ideas prior to dot voting. If for example, one idea was to "allow employees flex time within any given day – i.e., instead of 8 am–5 pm, allow 6 am until 3 pm" while another idea was to "allow flex time within any given pay period, i.e., eight-10-hour days versus 10-eight-hour days," the group may decide that these should be coupled into a single recommendation to "allow flex time."

Step 2: After combining or binning is complete and each idea represents an independent approach to the issue, number the remaining ideas in order. For the purposes of this illustration, we will say that 20 ideas remained.

Step 3: The facilitator gives each person an index card and tells them to write the numbers 1–20 consecutively from the top to the bottom of the card.

Step 4: The facilitator allocates the number of votes available and the most votes allowable for any one idea. This is derived using the method described in Box 3.5. This is not the only way to do this, but it has been found to be the best approach.

Step 5: Collect the votes and tally. Typically, two or three ideas dominate the voting. Some get no support and about half get weak support. This allows the group to concentrate on the best approaches to solving the problem. It is fairly easy to develop software that will automate this tool while preserving anonymity.

Box 3.5 Allocating Votes

Take the total number of ideas being considered (20), divide in half and add 1. This gives each person a total of 11 votes (if it were 19 ideas, just divide in "half" and give the larger number or 10).

Take this new number and allow a person to give 1/3 (rounded down) of their votes to any one idea. In this case it would be three votes.

Each person has a total of 11 votes to allocate against 20 ideas, and they can allocate a maximum number of three votes to any one idea (Fig. 3.4).

This approach does several things: It forces each person to prioritize in their own right while allowing them to express their passion for any one idea through a maximum allocation. However, it does not allow one person to dominate the voting by giving all 11 of their votes to their personal favorite.

Instruct participants to draw an "X" or check mark for each vote next to the number of the idea for which they are voting (i.e., if someone wanted to give three votes to idea number nine, they would write three "X's" next to the number nine).

Fig. 3.4 Allocating votes

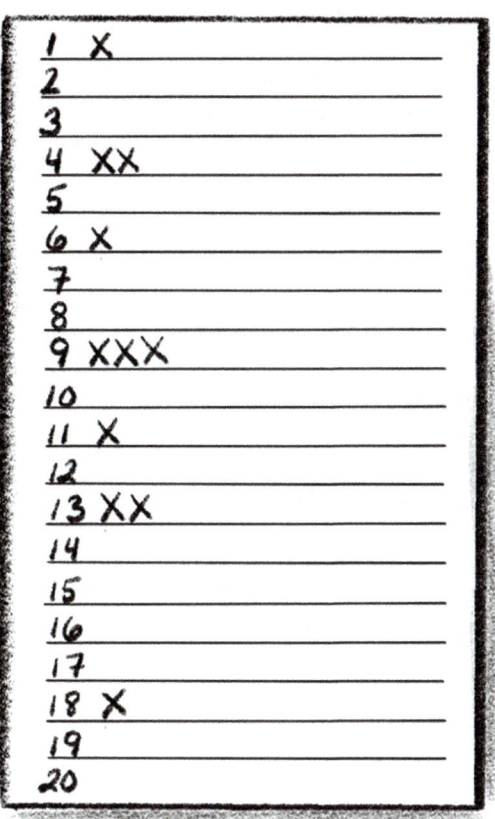

Forced Distribution

Forced distribution is simply a variant of *dot voting*. Instead of allocating a number of votes across a large number of options generated during divergence, this is a method best used when there are only a limited number of options generated (e.g., less than 10). This is also a good method if you want to avoid the prospect of any idea getting zero votes. This may happen if someone in the group is an outlier and highly sensitive. As illustration, let us assume there are 10 ideas generated. With *forced distribution*, participants are instructed that they must grade each idea anonymously on a scale of 1–10. However, they are limited to giving one-quarter of the votes scores of nine or ten, about half the votes scores between six and eight and one-quarter of the votes a five or below. In this way, every idea gets a score from everyone. In *dot voting,* some ideas risk getting no support other than that of the person who generated the idea.

Best of Breed

Best of Breed is a tool used in conjunction with *Ad Agency* (Chap. 4), but it can also be used independently. In *Ad Agency*, small groups of three each address a different element of the problem (e.g., whether to add a simulation center). Person One addresses the funding needed, Person Two addresses the need for more staffing, and Person Three addresses relevant space issues. They work together in the manner described in Chap. 4. After each team member has used the *Ad Agency* method, the *Best of Breed* approach is implemented. All Person Ones from each group gather together, as do all Person Twos and Person Threes to share the ideas they generated independently. Together, all Person Ones present their best ideas to the large group (everyone), determined either through discussion or *dot voting*. The Person Twos then present their group's best ideas followed by the Person Threes group.

Changing the Frame

Another set of Red Team tools used frequently are those whose underlying goal is to *change the frame* to make each individual think differently about their role and listen better to the contributions of others (Box 3.6).

Yes, and …

This tool is used to specifically counter the natural tendency to say "yes, but…." Among many groups, a competitive spirit develops among planners. This often results in people not listening well to each other's ideas. When one is talking, the other may be thinking about how to poke holes in or supplant the proposal with one of their own. *Yes,…and* is designed to force people to improve on each other's ideas instead of simply challenging them in a negative way. To use this tool, ask participants to state the other person's idea and add to it. This is similar to a children's game (that adults may also play) that starts with a few lines of a story. Each person in the game takes what was previously said and adds to the story. *Yes, and…* allows others to weigh in on the idea and attempt to improve it or challenge it. Routinely addressing each other in a *Yes, and…* manner can also help build a more cohesive and respectful team.

Box 3.6 Tools for Changing the Frame
- Yes and…
- My 15%.
- 4 ways of seeing.
- Role play.
- Second chance meeting.

A quick and simple illustration can demonstrate the power of this tool. If a group of people are assigned the task of planning an office party, but are told that as they listen to each other's suggestion they should say "yes, but," the conversation might go something like this:

- I recommend we have beer, wine, and an alcoholic punch to get everyone to really unwind
  - Yes, but people may get drunk and drive home
- I recommend we challenge each department to develop a skit
  - Yes, but a senior leader may get mad and it could have consequences for the skit team
- I recommend we hire a DJ to provide music
  - Yes, but not everyone has the same tastes and some music may offend some people

Compare this with the same conversation using a *yes,... and* approach:

- I recommend we have beer, wine, and an alcoholic punch to get everyone to really unwind
  - Yes, ... and we can solicit volunteers to run pick up and drop off services from among our staff that does not drink, or pay adult kids of staff to run the shuttles
- I recommend we challenge each department to develop a skit
  - Yes, ... and we can get prior approval for all skits from the associate dean so he/she takes the heat if anyone is offended
- I recommend we hire a DJ for music
  - Yes, ... and we can publish some guidelines on anything that is unacceptable. Yes, ... and we can invite each department to submit their own list of music. Yes, ... and we can build a rotation with the DJ that is both acceptable and represents the varied tastes of our staff

Adoption of a *yes,... and* instead of a *yes, but* culture can change an organization dramatically and replace roadblocks with imaginative problem solving.

My 15%

In every hierarchal organization, no matter how large or small, there is a tendency for those at the lower levels to believe that change must come from those above them. In reality, no one in any organization has complete control, but neither does anyone have zero control. We each control our own attitudes, personal priorities, time management, and how we engage with others. The intention of *my 15%* is to ask everyone to examine a problem through the perspective of what they can do without any additional resources, policy changes, or direction. Many human resource issues and professional development shortfalls can be addressed to some degree if those involved simply take a different look at the problem and ask, "what is my responsibility?" instead of "why don't my leaders fix this?" Philosophically, *my 15%* argues that "it is always better to light a candle, than curse the darkness." It is remarkable how often this simple approach can lead to real progress in solving a persistent issue.

4 Ways of Seeing

The *4 ways of seeing* (Table 3.1) is usually used in concert with *Stakeholder Analysis* which is described below. We will describe it first in the general case and then after explaining *Stakeholder Analysis,* explain how they are used together.

Whenever there are two people or organizations in dialogue, there are four different perspectives. There is the way X sees X; there is the way X sees Y; there is the way Y sees Y, and there is the way Y sees X. In our significant relationships, we know this intuitively. We know (and if we are smart, do not frequently voice) that our significant other, frequently sees their actions differently then we may see them. Just as we may see them differently than they see themselves, they in turn see us differently than our self-image. The object of *4 ways of seeing* is to think about these different perspectives in an organizational setting.

Nurses see themselves differently than nurses' aides see them. Just as nurses see physicians as a group differently than physicians see themselves. We will use these three groups to apply this method against a question. In this case, rather than the *4 ways of seeing*, it will become the "9 ways of seeing."

Problem: There is a new procedure associated with patient care that affects physicians, nurses, and nurses' aides.

The Method: *Step 1*: Designate the physicians as X, the nurses as Y, and nurses' aides as Z.

- *Step 2*: Create a 9-cell matrix with cell labels
    A. How physicians view the new procedure would be how X sees X.
    B. How physicians think nurses view the new procedure would be how X sees Y.
    C. How physicians think nurses' aides view the procedure is how X sees Z.
    D. How nurses see the new procedure would be how Y sees Y.
    E. How nurses think physicians see the new procedure would be how Y sees X.
    F. How nurses think aides see the procedure would be how Y sees Z.
    G. How nurses' aides view the new procedure would be how Z sees Z.
    H. How nurses' aides think physicians see the procedure would be how Z sees X.
    I. How nurses' aides think nurses see the procedure is how Z sees Y.

Table 3.1 4 ways of seeing

How X sees X	How Y sees Y
How X sees Y	How Y sees X

- *Step 3*: In an ideal world, this tool would be used by three different groups: physicians forming one group; nurses the second group, and nurses' aides, the third group. Whether in three groups or as a collective, address one cell at a time, using one of the liberating structures described above to collect the perspectives on the issue populating each cell.

For example, the *T-W-S* tool might be used initially so each person gets the opportunity to consider the issue at hand. Physicians as a group might think of the issue in one way while nurses and nurses' aides might have other perspectives. You can then ask the physicians (group X) to share together how they view the issue, how they think nurses (group Y) see the issue, and how they think nurses' aides (group Z) might view the issue. The nurses do the same about themselves, the physicians, and the nurses' aides. The nurses' aides do the same regarding the physicians and the nurses. Each group might then share these perspectives with the entire group of physicians, nurses, and nurses' aides.

Role Play

Telling a junior member of the staff that for the next small group discussion they will role play the Dean or the Chief Nurse is frequently fun and surprising. Those who normally have less power in an organization will be more likely to speak up if they have been assigned a powerful role by the facilitator. *Role play* can also be used to alter someone's perspective. If all of a sudden, the Director of Admissions needs to look at a problem as if they were the head of Information Technology, it will result in seeing things they otherwise would not. *Role play* is also embedded in tools like *AD Agency* described in Chap. 4.

Second Chance Meeting

After a group has used many of the other tools and struggled to develop a plan to address a problem, it is good practice to conduct a *second chance meeting*. Using this method, each member of the team is given an index card and asked anonymously to either endorse the proposed course of action or make their final objections. One of two outcomes is likely. First, everyone agrees with the plan. This is important because it binds everyone to publicly and privately endorsing the plan of action. The second outcome occurs when multiple people raise similar objections through their anonymous second chance. For example, 50% of the team might say the plan is great, but if it is just going to be added on to their already full workload with nothing removed, then they would never have time to properly implement it. This may lead to a second round of discussion focused on "what to stop doing" in order to implement the new approach.

Regular use of the tools in this chapter will change the culture of an organization. Everyone will get a chance to contribute. People will listen to each other more fully.

Ideas will prosper or perish based on the quality of the proposal. Individuals will begin to look for ways they can improve the organization in small ways and then share those ideas with others. These tools do not require a structured planning effort to merit implementation. Each reader can begin to use these tomorrow – where they work, live, and play.

The Red Team Tool Box: Understanding the Problem and Envisioning the Future

4

1. *Better understanding of the problem*: The golf club analogy in the Preface explained that if you do not understand the problem, you cannot choose the right club. The *Cynefin framework* and the 5 Whys are examples of tools that help us better understand the problem.
2. *Envisioning Alternative Futures (EAF)*: The tools used to envision alternative futures evolved in recognition that no matter how good a plan, the future has a way of emerging differently than anticipated. *Stakeholder mapping*, *TRIZ*, *Pre-mortem analysis*, *What-if analysis*, and *Ad Agency* are tools designed to help planners envision these futures before they occur so that as the future enfolds, we can remain agile in the execution of the plan.

Better Understanding the Problem

Cynefin Framework

A major challenge in problem identification is understanding the nature of the problem itself. The *Cynefin framework* is used to better understand the problem and how to address it. See Fig. 4.2.

The *Cynefin framework* divides the problem universe into four quadrants as described below:

1. *Simple problems*: For the purposes of this illustration, a simple problem is getting a copy of an old car key. We all remember how this was done: You went to a hardware store, brought in a copy of the key, selected a new key slug, and the hardware store employee put the slug and the old key on a machine and cut a new key. There is a clear best answer to how to solve this problem. No deep thinking is required and best practice is well established. We identify the problem, then use our knowledge of best practice to solve it. In the literature on *Cynefin*, this is known as *sense-categorize-respond*.

L. Neal-Boylan, S. Rotkoff, *Innovative Decision Making in Healthcare*,
https://doi.org/10.1007/978-3-030-72648-5_4

Fig. 4.1 Understanding
the problem and
envisioning the future.
(Drawings provided by
Tara J. Neal @
TaraNealArts)

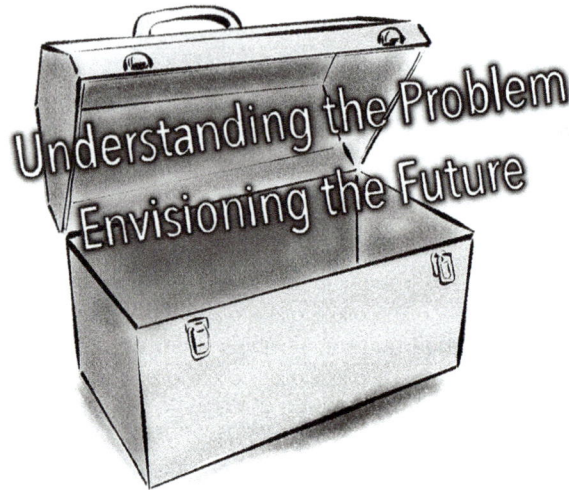

Fig. 4.2 Cynefin
framework

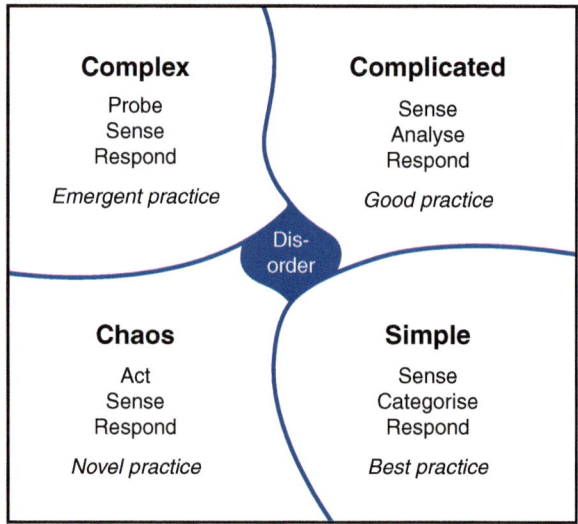

2. *Complicated problems*: To extend the example, this would be trying to build a
   car. Building a car is very complicated. It requires myriad parts, tools, and expertise. There may be more than one order in which to put the parts together.
   However, it can be described and laid out in detail and with enough time, tools,
   and expertise, it can be done and the end result will be roughly identical given
   the same parts and car model. This is harder to plan and execute than getting a
   new key to the car, but there are no unknowns about this process of building a car.

   Solving complicated problems: In this case while the problem is still defin-
   able, it requires some research. So, unlike a simple problem, a complicated one
   requires some analysis (review the schematics, get the right tools, etc.). Also

unlike the car key, there may be several good solutions to how to build the car. The analysis helps uncover the best solution in the given circumstance. *Cynefin framework* refers to this as *sense-analyze-respond*.

3. *Complex problems*: An example of this is driving a car to work each day. Even if you are driving on your daily commute and the route is identical, the problem is complex. The weather changes, a kid can run out into the street, and there are detours and delays. It is never completely the same twice.

   Solving complex problems: Complex problems require continuous engagement during the problem (driving) solving process. The problem is solved only when you get to the end of the issue; problem solutions emerge over time. Addressing these problems requires that you, *probe-sense-respond*. As you conduct the drive, you are doing so in a controlled manner probing the environment by moving the car forward in a predetermined way. You pay close attention for kids playing in the street and you respond as necessary to your probes by adjusting your driving.

4. *Chaotic problems*: An example of this would be our driver being caught in the middle of a shootout in a foreign country and having to seize the wheel and drive for the first time on the opposite side of the road, unable to read the traffic signs, while someone is shooting at them.

   Addressing chaotic problems: These problems are not solved. The situation requires you to act first, then figure out what comes next. In the scenario above, failure to act means you will be shot. For these kinds of issues, we *act-sense-respond*. In our example, this would be to drive like a madman to get out of the situation, notice that you are driving on the wrong side of the road, notice that you are away from the crime scene, and respond by slowing down or pulling over.

Addressing the right problem is also necessary to begin using Red Teaming tools. The *5 Whys* can help determine the root cause.

The 5 Whys

The *5 Whys* was originally developed by the Toyota Corporation. It resulted from repeated attempts to fix elements of the assembly line for car production. After some investigation, the leaders in Toyota learned that the repairs they were performing did not address the root cause of the problem. Rather, it was an entirely different element of the assembly line that was, over time, causing the specific part they had been replacing to wear out. Until they addressed the root cause, they would continue to replace faulty elements that were downstream in the assembly line from the root cause of the problem.

The *5 Whys* method does not always require five full rounds of inquiry; however, years of use across a variety of professions have resulted in the adoption of this name, since most root causes can be identified within five rounds of questioning. Start with the problem:

Problem   Nurses are not universally using gloves to perform wound care

- Why 1 – Why are nurses not universally using gloves?
- Answer – Some nurses who do not always use gloves say when they wear gloves, they lose tactile ability to perform some functions.
- Why 2 – Why are these nurses losing tactile function when wearing gloves?
- Answer – They frequently cannot find the right-sized gloves; gloves that are too large (the usual case) are not snug enough to provide good tactile control.
- Why 3 – Why can't they find gloves that are the right size?
- Answer – Glove stocks frequently run out of small-sized gloves.
- Why 4 – Why are glove stocks not constantly supplied with all sizes of gloves?
- Answer – There is no systematic approach to ensuring glove stocks are refilled based on usage.
- Why 5 – Why are glove stocks not being monitored systematically?
- Answer – No one has been assigned the responsibility to monitor and fill glove stocks.

The advantage of the *5 Whys* is that you solve the real problem. The problem is not that nurses do not want to wear gloves. In fact, they are not wearing gloves only when it interferes with patient care. The real problem in this illustration is the system for monitoring and restocking gloves and who owns that responsibility. If the root cause is fixed – glove availability – then the symptomatic problem of occasional non-use of gloves is solved.

Distinguishing the Problem to Be Solved

It is important to distinguish among the different kinds of problems being solved. Let us use the recent COVID 19 pandemic as an example. When the crisis started, it was clearly a chaotic problem, with healthcare workers acting first and assessing the efficacy of their actions over a number of trials. As more was learned, it became a complex problem with no predetermined end date. Once treatment protocols, contact tracing, and universal testing became available, it transitioned to a complicated problem. Now that we have an effective vaccine, it is a simple problem.

When the nature of the problem is misunderstood by leaders, it can result in dysfunctional guidance. For example, once transmission and symptoms were well understood, those advising consideration of untested actions to prevent or cure the virus were acting as if it was a chaotic problem long after it had become a complicated one. Similarly, those disregarding the need for masks, or claiming the virus will simply go away, treated the virus as a simple problem when it still remained complicated. Thus, the approach was not appropriate for the stage of problem solving.

Envisioning Alternative Futures

1. *Stakeholder mapping* (Fig. 4.3). When trying to introduce any new approach, it is first necessary to identify who in the organization is invested in the status quo, and why they hold their opinion. Red Teaming uses two tools in tandem to better understand the organizational playing field when bringing new ideas forward. They are *Stakeholder Mapping* and *4 ways of seeing* (see Chap. 3)

Use one of the divergence tools (Chap. 3) to liberate the conversation and generate the widest collection of invested stakeholders.

Step 1: Use a *liberating structure* to capture all of the stakeholders invested in the issue at hand. For example, in an academic setting, this might include the director of the baccalaureate in nursing program, faculty who teach in that program, baccalaureate nursing students, and the secretary who supports that program. At this stage, you do not care if they are likely to be in favor, opposed, or neutral about the proposed new idea. Once you have collected all stakeholders, assign numbers to them.

Step 2: This step can be done anonymously, but does not have to be. Rank the stakeholders based on how critical their participation is in order to implement the new idea. There may be stakeholders whom the change will affect, but have little influence on implementation and there may be stakeholders without whom the new idea cannot be implemented. At this stage, defer assessing whether the stakeholder is supportive or opposed to the idea. The only question is how necessary each one is to idea implementation. Those who are very necessary are ranked at 10; those unnecessary for implementation are ranked at 1, with gradations in between.

Fig. 4.3 Stakeholder mapping

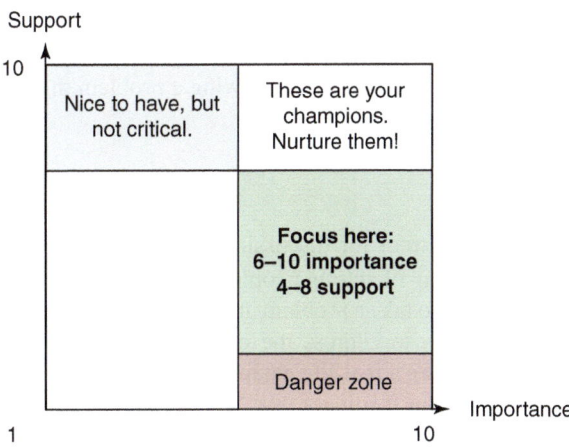

Step 3: Evaluate if these stakeholders are supportive or opposed to the idea. Those very supportive are a 10; those very non-supportive are a 1, again, with gradations in between.

Step 4: Map the stakeholders on a graph. Along the X-axis, place a 1 on the far left; place a 10 on the far right. Along the Y-axis, the bottom number should be a 1 and the top number should be a 10. Label the X-axis "level of support" for the new approach; label the Y-axis "level of importance" to implementation. Thus, the most important and most supportive stakeholders are listed (by number) in the upper right quadrant.

Step 5: Identify those stakeholders who require the most attention to influence them to support the proposal. These stakeholders generally fall between the 6–10 range on the "importance to implementation" scale and the 3–7 range on their "level of support." The focus of the *4 ways of seeing* tool is on this group. (NOTE: if you have a stakeholder who is a 9–10 on "level of importance" and a 1–3 on "level of support," you should question the viability of pursuing the issue being discussed).

Let us now apply the *4 ways of seeing* illustration. Using this problem: There is a new procedure associated with patient care that affects nurses, physicians, and nurses' aides. It cannot be emphasized enough how the simple process of trying to see an issue through the eyes of different groups can be revelatory. While physicians and nurses may love this new process, since it makes their lives easier, nurses' aides may be thoroughly against it. If they are the critical factor (based on stakeholder analysis) in implementing the procedure, then a strategy needs to be developed targeting them as a group. Either they need to be convinced of the need for the new procedure, or the procedure needs to be modified to accommodate their issues. Identifying the key stakeholders, culling out the ones who must be convinced, taking the time to understand their issues, and then developing a strategy to address those issues are processes that, while appearing obvious, are often overlooked during the introduction of new methods in organizations. This tool has proven to be very effective in stimulating viewing a problem through multiple perspectives.

TRIZ

This is a fun tool for discussing difficult topics. It was developed in the Soviet Union as a way of getting people to tell difficult truths without retribution. The idea of the tool is to take a problem and design the *worst* possible set of processes, policy, behavior, etc., to address the problem to *ensure failure* of the system. It is best explained using a real-life example:

A Red Team facilitator was brought into an organization to lead a series of Red Teaming methods to discuss a university's long-range plan. During a break, the president of the university approached the facilitator and told him that he had reports that one of his key staff had recently insulted him in public when he was not present. He wanted to address the issue, but he did not want to call her out by name or create more friction in his small (seven) leadership team.

After returning from the break, the facilitator broke the group (the president, his executive secretary, and his seven subordinate leaders, totaling nine) into three sub-groups of three. The facilitator explained to the group that there were three important ways that they communicated:

- Behind closed doors among the nine of them
- In sub-groups of the leadership team, typically two or three talking independently of the other members
- With other people in the university who were not part of the leadership team

The facilitator assigned each group of three to examine one of the three types of communication outlined above. The charge for each group was to design rules that would guarantee failure of the leadership team over all, and that would fuel dissension and distrust.

The outcome of this effort was fabulous. As each group briefed the others, they played with the tool, identifying a huge number of things that would collectively hurt them. Finally, they acknowledged that they already were doing some of the things identified. The final outcome was that they collectively wrote a leadership team code of conduct that they all signed. They anonymously affirmed their acceptance of the new code of conduct using a *second chance meeting*. This code of conduct has guided them since and has vastly improved their group dynamics. The woman who insulted the president is still part of the team, much better behaved and completely oblivious that the tool was introduced because of her behavior.

Pre-mortem Analysis

This tool is designed to stress-test a plan. Without, as a minimum, the broad outline of a plan, this tool cannot be effectively used. This tool was invented by Gary Klein [1] who was introduced in Chap. 2, but we have adapted it through repeated experimentation to be more than his original design. As the name *pre-mortem* implies, the tool is used to help people imagine failure of the plan in order to build in metrics and mitigation strategies to avoid failure in execution. (The word post-mortem typically refers to reviewing a plan after it has already failed).

Most planning begins from the current state and moves forward to the desired future state using the plan as a way to get to that better future. *Pre-mortem analysis* is unique in that it reverses the process of our thinking. It starts with a future failed state and asks us to imagine ways in which the plan could go wrong that led to that failure. It fundamentally changes the way we think about the problem, plan, and alternative futures. This is by far, the most popular and widely used tool in the Red Teaming collection.

Step 1: There must be some outline of a plan: We intend to accomplish the following thing in the following way over the following time period.

Step 2: Each person on the team needs to individually imagine a future where the plan they are developing has failed in a dramatic way. The cause of this failure may be anything, as long as it is realistic and possible within the time frame identified in step 1.

Step 3: Once future failure has been imagined and described (what does the organization look like now that we have failed?), each person has to build a backward timeline that explains the events that led to the failure – that timeline should lead from the time of failure until today.

Step 4: Once everyone has prepared their individual pre-mortems, they are shared with the entire group.

Step 5: Everyone is asked to look for common events or themes across the individually developed pre-mortems. Frequently, there are common events that occurred leading to different kinds of failure. For example, a data breach leaking the private information of donors can lead to financial failure with accounts being hacked, can lead to a public relations failure, or could lead to a failure to attract future donors. All of these failure scenarios would be different, but the common element would be the data hack that contributed to all three.

Step 6: Using some *liberating structures*, look for ways to *PRECLUDE* the event from happening, *MONITOR* warning signs that the event is happening, and *REACT* if the event happens.

The following is an example of how to use this tool. Jane and John have built a plan to retire with financial security by the age of 65. They have spent a lot of energy capturing their monthly expenses and thinking about what they need for their retirement income and looking at investment options. They are pretty happy with their plan but decide to conduct a mini-*pre-mortem* analysis. They follow the steps as described below:

Step 1: They have a plan.

Step 2: They each individually envision the failure of their plan.

Step 3: They walk that failure back until the present day, describing the imagined events that led to failure.

Step 4: They share their pre-mortems with each other:

In Jane's pre-mortem, they cannot retire because they have a series of unexpected expenses associated with their aging parents that forces them to continue working. Her pre-mortem looks like this:

- We cannot retire because our parents need financial assistance due to health and personal care considerations.
- Our parents needed help because they did not plan for their own financial longevity challenges.
- We did not have enough because in our plan we assumed they would remain self-sufficient.

In John's pre-mortem, they cannot retire because they simply did not meet their financial contribution goals over the years. His pre-mortem looks like this:

- We cannot retire because we have unexpected expenses each year that have decremented our contributions.
- We have car replacement, roof repair, wedding costs, etc. These are not reflected in our budget.
- We assumed our miscellaneous category was big enough and did not visualize some of the truly large expenses we might encounter.

Step 5: The common theme is that they cannot retire because of a variety of different kinds of unexpected expenses that derail their plan.

Step 6: Preclude

- Jane and John will ask their parents to buy long-term care insurance. If they are unwilling or cannot afford to do so, John and Jane will buy it for them. Buying it now enables John and Jane to have some security regarding their parents' future expenses and can be built into their budget.

Monitor
- Jane and John will redo their budget with a larger portion of their investments in "cash-like" instruments that allow them both to invest but also be able to respond rapidly to unexpected needs. They will keep a record each month to better capture these "unexpected events" and revise their overall budget accordingly

React
- If necessary, they are prepared to extend their working lives until age 68 and retire earlier only if it becomes possible.

Pre-mortem With and Without Liberating Structures

As described in the Preface and again in Chap. 2, Red Team methods and liberating structures are meta-ideas. The description above is pre-mortem with the incorporation of LS through use of *TWS*. Below for comparison purposes is an illustration of Pre-mortem without LS.

The team leader asks everyone to imagine failure of the plan and things that would have caused that failure. The leader does not set aside time for everyone in the group to individually develop their pre-mortem so people start shouting out ideas in an undisciplined way. Those who are less confident or less senior simply say that another member of the team shared their idea already. While the intent of the tool is the same, the mechanics are entirely different. Lacking a LS to ensure everyone's thoughtful participation, the results are much less creative or helpful to the planning process.

What-If Analysis

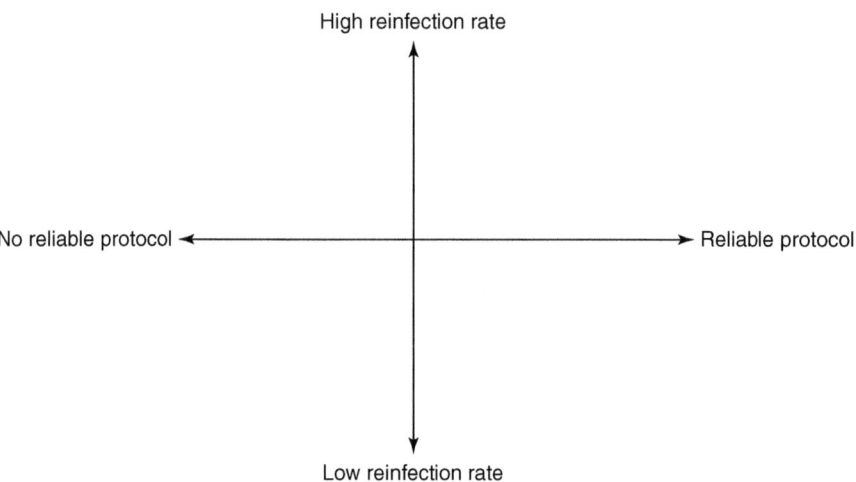

This tool is also known as scenario planning and is a staple of business programs. Like stakeholder analysis, this tool uses a four box X–Y-axis approach.

Step 1: Identify two independent variables about a problem that can have a range of future outcomes. In most cases (but not all, these are linked to some timeline).

For illustration, we will use the graph shown above. The X-axis will represent the development of protocols for treatment for COVID-19 using a time frame of less than 12 months. On the left side of the X-axis, protocols are still not fully understood and treatments rely on educated guesses versus routinized procedures (no reliable protocol). On the right side of the X-axis, there is a well-tested approach to treating specific patients (reliable protocol). The Y-axis reflects the status of reinfection of those who have already had the virus. The top of the Y-axis reflects a high reinfection rate and the bottom of the Y-axis is close to a 0 reinfection rate.

This posits four very different futures. In the bottom left quadrant, protocols are limited and reinfection rates are high. Consequently, continued social distancing, continued production of ventilators, and masking are absolutely imperative.

In the top right quadrant, protocols are well established, but reinfection rate is high. This becomes a supply chain problem: Having the right equipment based on good data about the nature of the infected population, coupled with good data on the best way to treat patients.

In the bottom left quadrant, protocols are limited, but reinfection is also limited. Those who have been infected and recovered can return to work. The key is voluminous testing to separate the already infected from the not yet infected.

Finally in the bottom right quadrant, protocols are well established and reinfection is close to zero – this is when getting back to normal is most possible.

This simple but elegant tool enables us to think of four different futures, collect data to see which is emergent in fact, and then be best prepared to act as it does.

Ad Agency

The purpose of this tool is to foster several effective Red Teaming methods simultaneously. First, it puts everyone into a *yes,...and* frame of mind. Second, it begins with small groups and aggregates upward fostering creative solutions, and finally it results in looking at the same problem through a variety of different lens.

This tool is called *Ad Agency* because it requires two of the three-person small group to act as an advertising agency, hearing the ideas of the third person. The third member of the group serves as the client, so the agency must take a *yes,...and* attitude toward their ideas. If they criticize instead of improving upon an idea, they risk losing the client.

This tool works best when there are three separate, but related aspects of the plan being developed or the problem to be solved, or if there are three different approaches under consideration. For the purposes of this illustration, the challenge is cutting school expense costs. The group has developed three approaches. The planning team is then divided into groups of three (Person A, Person B, and Person C), with each person in the group assigned responsibility for a different one of the three ways (options A, B, or C) being considered (each group of three has all three ideas represented in their group).

Step 1: Each person is directed that they *MUST* design a smart approach to reducing expenditures in their assigned area. They cannot debate the wisdom of doing so, they must imagine they have been directed to do so and must then design the best way to implement the approach to save the most money with the least impact on revenue generation and quality of education.

Step 2: Each person in each team works to design their approach independently without consultation of the other team members.

Step 3: Once each person has designed their plan, they sit in a small circle with the other two team members. The advocate for reducing travel reimbursement (Person A) speaks first. The other two members who serve as the *Ad Agency* listen and take notes. After Person A has finished their presentation, they walk away and give the Ad Agency time to talk about their proposal.

Step 4: The *Ad Agency*, consisting of the remaining team members (persons B and C), must find ways to improve, instead of rebut or dismiss Person A's proposal. Like an advertising agency, they cannot tell the client he/she is wrong or ignorant; instead, they must build on and improve the client's ideas. They consult with each other first without the client present so they can speak openly about the ideas and consider how to improve them.

Step 5: The client (Person A) returns to the *Ad Agency* and listens to the team's feedback on how to improve the idea. The client asks questions to understand their feedback and takes notes.

Steps 3–5 are then repeated with team members B and C designated as the advocates for options B and C, respectively. Person B plays the client through steps 3–5 followed by Person C as the client.

Step 6: The teams now separate into the committee members who represented each option. The committee members representing option A (all Person A's) get together and build a list of the best option A ideas to save money with the least impact. Persons B get together and Persons C get together. Each team builds a *best of breed* list to give to the entire group.

Step 7: Representatives from options A, B, and C present their proposals in turn, to the entire committee.

Step 8: The committee members vote for the best ideas within options A, B, and C using the *dot voting* technique (see Chap. 3).

This chapter does *NOT* describe the complete universe of tools available to the Red Team practitioner. In fact, that would be impossible to do. Once you become comfortable with these tools you will find yourself creating your own tools based on the same principles but tailored to the specific need to the problem you are addressing. In 15 years of facilitating Red Teams, author SR has used literally 100 tools. Some he designed on the fly and used only once. The group included in this chapter reflects the tried and true and most frequently used tools. Do not be afraid to create your own. Remember, divergence before convergence, anonymity leads to truth, and the future will always be emergent.

Reference

1. Klein GA. Sources of power: how people make decisions. Cambridge, MA: MIT Press; 1999. ISBN 0-262-61146-5.

Applying Red Team Tools

5

It is helpful to think of Red Teaming as a set of recipes. For example: There are many types of recipes/tools with which to make a great chocolate chip cookie, and all include some fundamental ingredients that play certain roles, but those ingredients can change: granulated sugar vs. agave, all-purpose flour vs. almond flour, etc. As a Red Teamer, the job is to understand the demands of the situation and the audience. At what altitude are we baking? Do we have vegan friends coming over? Does the dough need to be refrigerated before baking? A skilled Red Teamer will become good enough to become more creative with their recipes. (Maple bacon chocolate chip cookies, perhaps?).

Like baking, there are some underlying guides, but no fixed rules, and the best bakers adjust to their circumstances. Thus, there are no set forms or formats for how to Red Team, the very notion is anathema to the underlying precepts.

As discussed briefly in the Preface, the downside of fixed methods like Lean Six Sigma [1] are that filling in the steps to complete the "methodology" quickly becomes the goal of the planning group. Ultimately, slavish adherence to methods stands in the way of original thought. Red Teaming is designed to encourage innovation and original thought. The methodology involved is intended to be a guide and adaptable to the context and circumstances. The Preface briefly introduced the five steps of a generic Red Team methodology. This chapter will take a closer look into each of those steps. Assume the leader has presented a problem, issue, or question to the Red Team. Box 5.1 lists the steps to follow.

It is important to further deconstruct the steps of this process.

© The Author(s), under exclusive license to Springer Nature Switzerland AG 2021   47
L. Neal-Boylan, S. Rotkoff, *Innovative Decision Making in Healthcare*,
https://doi.org/10.1007/978-3-030-72648-5_5

Box 5.1 Steps Required to Red Team

- *Step 1 – Take time to understand the root problem –* One can use *Cynefin*, the *5 whys, anonymous feedback,* or other Red Team tools, but make sure to identify and solve the right underlying issue.
- *Step 2 –* Understand the time available for the Red Team, the audience for the Red Team, the people who will compose the Red Team, and the *circumstances under which the Red Team will be conducted.*
- *Step 3 –* Once it is clear, the right issue is being reviewed and the constraints are understood, *pick those tools most suited to that SPECIFIC circumstance.*
- *Step 4 – Red Team.*
- *Step 5 – Present the results.*

Step 1: Understand the Root Problem

The biggest hurdle in addressing any issue is making sure the team understands the underlying root cause of the problem. Frequently, organizations are thrown into crisis planning because some important metric is under-performing. In an academic institution for example, donor contributions, enrollments, or grants may not be meeting the expected standard. Typically, the initial instinct is to simply ramp up already existing efforts. For example, make another plea to reliable donors or reach out to new ones, step up recruitment, or write more grants. While none of these approaches are flawed, they do not address the fundamental "why" question. Why are there fewer donor contributions? If the answer is a general downturn in the economy, then perhaps the best strategy is to tell donors we are also tightening our belts and ask for a small donation to keep them connected to our school until the economy improves, when we will ask them for more. If, however, they are donating less because of some new school policy or adverse publicity, then our approach must be completely different to bring them back into the fold. Similar illustrations can be made for any underperforming metric we hope to address. Thus, the first and most important step to set the Red Team on the path to success is understanding "why."

Before moving on, it is worth taking a moment to ask: If asking "why" is so important, then why do organizations default to doing what they have always done? The reason may have to do with risk. If one advocates for doing more of what the organization is already doing and with which they are comfortable, there is no associated risk. Advocating for a reexamination of why one is failing to meet goals may challenge ideas with which the organization is comfortable and hold dear. The business landscape is littered with stories of successful organizations that refused to challenge their way of doing business and never examined the "why" question. Famously, the Polaroid company realized they were starting to lose a minor amount of market share to digital cameras. Unfortunately, they were so entrenched in their culture of selling and processing film, they never asked themselves why. Consequently, despite inventing the digital camera they eventually went out of business entirely.

Another element of understanding the problem deals with whether it is simple, complicated, complex, or chaotic (Chap. 4). Diagnosing the nature of the problem is much like what a nurse practitioner does when diagnosing a patient. The same symptoms (coughing, sneezing, difficulty breathing, etc.) may signify a relatively benign etiology, such as an allergy or it may mean something more serious, such as COVID 19. The diagnostician figures out how to treat the patient by asking questions and running tests to better understand the nature of the problem. Understanding the problem is not curing the problem – that requires some form of treatment. In the same way, the *Cynefin framework* helps the planning team understand the nature of the project or problem they must address. The Red Team facilitator can determine which tools to use once the root cause and fundamental nature of the problem are understood.

Step 2: Red Team Circumstances

The circumstances under which the Red Team will be operating is another key consideration in determining which tools to use.

Choosing the Team

The nursing profession is a big proponent of inclusivity and diversity. However, we tend to define diversity in terms of gender identity, ethnicity, age, and similar factors. But the goal of diversity in any planning or decision-making group is diversity of thought. To achieve diversity of thought, the training, education, and experience of those in the room can frequently count as much, or more, than ethnicity, gender, or other markers of diversity. A group of nurses may look very diverse from the outside, but if they have all been taught to think in terms of adherence to best practices, they may not really be diverse in their thinking. (It is helpful to note that the Titanic was built in accordance with all of the best engineering practices of the time). If most people in the group have a nursing education, add someone with an undergraduate degree in fine arts or music to the Red Team.

This is not to suggest that knowledge of the issue is unimportant. It would not be possible for a group of plumbers to Red Team the management of patients coming to an emergency room. However, if the entire team consists of people who have spent the bulk of their careers working in emergency rooms, look for at least one generalist to join the team. The generalist will question things the group takes for granted. If the person who is different from the others in the group is fundamentally smart and a good team player, the time taken to teach this person the fundamentals of the problem will be well worth the insight and challenge they bring to the team.

Another analogy may help describe team composition. If the object of the Red Team were to examine and revise curricula, the optimal Red Team would not consist exclusively of experts in curriculum design. While some members of the team should be curriculum experts, they should be complemented by faculty with expertise in each of the courses to be reviewed and revised, someone from academic support, the associate dean of academic affairs, and perhaps the assistant dean of student affairs.

If composing and conducting a Red Team in the organization is not a bit painful, then it is a waste of time. The people who comprise the Red Team cannot be those who have the most availability to participate. If the Red Team is not composed of quality people with some bona fides, the results of the effort will not be well received.

A Red Teamer must be a good communicator. The team as a group, must have high quality oral, written, and graphic communication abilities. Fundamentally, a Red Team is utilized to tell someone there are aspects of their plan or decision that can be improved. This requires finesse and empathy. Nurses are experts at empathy. Empathy is one of the most important characteristics of quality Red Teamers. Empathy, not sympathy, is necessary to see things from another's perspective, whether they are a stakeholder, a competitor, or a typically under-valued member of one's team or organization.

Choosing the Time

Typically, half a day is the minimum time needed to Red Team anything worth the effort. Whenever possible, it is ideal to use 2–3 days consisting of 4 hours each. Red Teaming is most effective when given sufficient time; however, time between Red Teaming is important because the discussion within the Red Team will percolate in each team member's subconscious during the space between engagements. The results are frequently much better as a consequence.

Assume the leader or boss has presented a plan to the Red Team. It is possible to conduct an *Abbreviated Red Team* (Box 5.2) for 4 hours on a single day, but that limits

---

Box 5.2 Red Teaming for Three, Four-Hour Days
1. The first 4 hours utilize *Abbreviated Red Team*:
   - Spend some time understanding the "why" of the issue at hand.
   - Utilize some form of divergence to collect anonymous feedback from the team on the most pressing problems.
   - Preliminary discussions on the underlying assumptions that must be true for the plan to be realized and what to do if those assumption prove false.
2. The next 4 hours use *liberating structures* and an appropriate tool (such as *Ad Agency*) to develop mitigation strategies around those issues identified in the first 4 hours.
3. The final 4 hours usually deal with *envisioning alternative futures* through tools such as *what-if analysis* or *pre-mortem analysis* and then developing warning signs or metrics to alert the team if negative alternative futures begin to emerge, along with associated mitigation strategies.

the tools one can realistically use; the team MUST spend some time understanding the "why" of the issue at hand. Once the "why" is understood, Red Teaming must utilize some form of divergence to collect anonymous feedback from the team on the most pressing problems with the plan. If time allows, there should be some preliminary discussions on the underlying assumptions that must be true for the plan (as initially provided by the leader or boss) to be realized and what to do if the plan's assumptions prove false. It is unrealistic to expect more from a half-day of Red Teaming.

It is highly preferable to conduct two or three concurrent days of 4 hours each versus one 8–12-hour Red Team. Red Teaming is mentally tiring, and some tools are best conducted individually at home over a glass of wine. However, sometimes it is logistically impossible to stretch out the team effort if people have traveled a long distance to participate. In that case, make sure to build in long breaks for people to refresh and reflect during the event. Additionally, concurrent days are preferred because the team may lose what has already been accomplished if meetings are separated by long periods of time. Box 5.2 describes an example of Red Teaming conducted during 3, 4-hour days.

The timeline in Box 5.2 does not include the time required to rehearse the presentation following the Red Team exercises. This is also a critical event. If the Red Team recommendations are valuable, then there is a good chance that some of them may be controversial. Time spent figuring out how to tell the leader or boss their plan has flaws is just as important as the time spent identifying the flaws.

It is important to note that there is no set time required for Red Teaming. A large Fortune 100 company devoted a full week of strategic planning time to a single high-value initiative. Red Teaming takes time. It is intended to take time. By its very nature, it slows down the rush to decide quickly, in order to create thinking space for individual and group reflection.

Choosing the Space and Supplies

Ambiance counts! Wherever possible, avoid Red Teaming in a sterile room with no windows, poor lighting, or limited room to move. Many of the tools require the group to break into small teams or to move around. Additionally, an institutional feel to the space reinforces institutional thinking. Meeting off campus in a room with picture windows allows the mind to wander. Box 5.3 lists the contents of a Red Teaming "kit" to be used during in-person Red Teaming. Box 5.4 lists the contents of the Red Team workbook. Box 5.5 lists tools needed if Red Teaming is conducted online.

Knowing the Audience and the Role of "Tone"

It is impossible to conduct an effective Red Team presentation or out-briefing without knowing the audience along with any office politics surrounding the issue being addressed. There is a vast difference between analyzing the problem effectively and developing useful feedback and feedback that is "heard" by the leaders to whom the

Box 5.3 Tools of the Trade
1. A stack of colored 8 × 11 index cards. These enable *5 will get you 25* in the most effective way. Also, index cards can be used at the end of each day to provide *anonymous feedback* to the facilitator on the quality of that day's activities along with suggestions for the next day.
2. Either a room surrounded with white boards including erasable markers or a large number of "butcher-paper" pads that can stand on easels. These are critical for small group work.
3. A single style of pens in large enough quantities to equip all members of the team with the same implement. This can become an important component of maintaining anonymity.
4. A tailored workbook that includes a description of all of the tools the facilitator intends to use with the team (see Box 5.4).

Box 5.4 Workbook Table of Contents
1. The purpose of the Red Team meetings.
2. The rules of engagement among the group and the tools/approaches to be used during the Red Team meetings.
3. A brief narrative about the "why" and history of Red Team tools and application.
4. The analyzed data received prior to the start of the Red Team meetings, to include the scoring of priorities received from the person or persons who called for Red Teaming the issue. Additionally, any data regarding any known differences between the staff and the leadership regarding the issue at hand, should be included.

Box 5.5 Online Red Teaming "Kit"
1. An ability to rapidly break into sub-rooms and then return to the large group.
2. Automated tools designed to enable anonymity.
3. The ability to build spreadsheets to use tools, such as *dot voting*.

Red Team results are presented. Box 5.6 lists some questions the Red Team should ask itself before presenting their recommendations.

This is not to suggest that the Red Team shape their feedback to what the audience wants to hear. Doing so would nullify the purposes of having a Red Team. This is to alert those participating in Red Teams that tone matters. The people who developed the plan, question, or project that was Red Teamed never intended to do something flawed. They worked hard on their plan or project and at some level, they all hope the Red Team will report that their plan is perfect! There are several tried and true strategies for delivering bad news to the project leader or the boss in a way that makes it easier for them to hear (Box 5.7).

> **Box 5.6 Questions for the Red Team**
> - What are the roles and relationships among those who will attend the presentation?
> - Who was the advocate for Red Teaming? Why did they advocate for Red Teaming? What is the underlying motive that drove the decision to Red Team this project/plan/problem/question?
> - Is there anyone in the room who is liable to lose their job or be professionally embarrassed by our feedback?
> - Is there anyone in the room inclined to be our ally, based on our proposed findings?
> - How does the decision-maker in the room best process information? For example, by oral presentation, written paper, or open conversation?
> - How will the organization or boss define "success" of this Red Teaming effort?

> **Box 5.7 Delivering Bad News to the Person or Team That Proposed the Original Idea, Plan, Question, or Project**
> - *Maybe we failed to understand*: This method allows the receiver to consider the possibility that their original plan is fine, simply unclear.
> - *We can tell how much work you have put into this. You have been so close to it, there appears to be some things that you may have become blind to due to your immersion*: The team erred because it was working so hard it became "blind" to some aspects of the plan. Again, this approach gives the team that wrote the plan an out for what they have overlooked.
> - *The underlying concept of this plan is brilliant; we have some comments around the margins*: Compliment, then criticize; this is a time-honored way of providing feedback that is difficult to hear.

Step 3: Tools Suited to the Circumstance

Never allow the tools described in this book to become sacrosanct in their implementation. All tools can and should be adjusted to the particulars of the Red Team. Below are examples of how Red Team tools were adapted to fit the situation.

Use of Role Play: In a real-life Red Team scenario, all members of the Red Team were senior or formerly senior military officers. Building and encouraging diversity of thought inside such a group was a challenge. The facilitator came up with a unique approach. For the initial review of the policy in question, each member of the Red Team was assigned a specific perspective that was not their own. One reviewed the policy from the perspective of our allies, the other from our adversaries, another from the likely perspective of congressional Republicans, another from that of

Democrats; the perspectives of the media and the national security academic community were also included. Each member of the Red Team was given time to research their assigned character's perspective on the issues and then review the policy through the lenses associated with their role. The result was a wide variety of ideas in a room in which the similarity of experiences and education of the group would normally have led to groupthink.

Building the Competitors Case: One of the companies with whom this author (SR) worked was getting ready to put a very large investment into a new public initiative. They knew from experience that their prime competitor would develop a counter campaign. Because this was a technical firm, they tended to think in terms of the capabilities of their product and how their competitor would counter from a capability perspective. SR asked the Red Team to become their own competitor for a few hours. He bought them their competitor's t-shirts and had them wear them during the exercise. His charter to the team was to come up with the most damaging counter campaign possible. The result was dynamite! The team attacked the verbiage and promised deliverables of the new product in a way that demeaned the proposed new capability. Rather than focus on the technical specifics, they started to think like their competitor who was always very good at creating belittling memes aimed at their company. As a consequence of this Red Team, the company decided to completely change the branding of their product to remove their vulnerability to sarcasm or insult that would likely have resulted from the first approach.

Neither of the two methods described above are standard Red Team methods. They were both designed around the specifics of the problem, audience, and time available. Note also that both of them included an element of role play. Role play is enormously effective if the right roles are assigned. This will always be a tool that requires tailoring to the issue, the team, and the circumstances.

Step 4: Red Team Roles

There are several key functions that need to be conducted to ensure an orderly and useful Red Team effort. If circumstances require, these functions can be performed by as few as two people: The Red Team facilitator and the note taker.

Red Team Facilitator

The person in the facilitator role should understand the Red Team tools and be neutral regarding the topic to be discussed. Their job is facilitating versus advocating. If the group construes that the facilitator is an advocate for a specific outcome, then the Red Team effort will lose all credibility within the team. However, the facilitator can comment, question, or clarify findings. This is appropriate.

However, the findings should originate with the team, not the facilitator. An important role of the facilitator is to sense when the group is going off topic or retreading old ground. The facilitator keeps the team moving forward, giving enough time for weighty issues to be discussed, but helping the group avoid flailing or bogging down. This skill is as much art as science and like Red Teaming itself, facilitators get better with practice.

Also, the Red Team facilitator must continually sense what is happening with the Red Team participants. Are there conflicts arising between specific members? Are there team members who are being drowned out because their ideas are too contrarian? Are there skills and insights among the team that are not being leveraged? The facilitator constantly "takes the temperature" of the team and makes adjustments, as necessary, to leverage the contributions of all team members and prevent fractious in-fighting among the team.

Note Taker

The note taker is the second necessary position on any Red Team. It is not possible to effectively facilitate and also take notes. Recording Red Team sessions is possible if the team is comfortable with that option. One of the prime functions of the note taker is to separate the wheat from the chaff. A rich conversation is the normal by-product of the use of Red Team tools. It is the job of the note taker to listen carefully and capture all the critical nuggets as they are revealed. This is not a job for a stenographer who records discussions verbatim, rather it is for an informed and engaged member of the team who listens well and has a talent for synopsizing discussions.

Timekeeper

The timekeeping function can be conducted by the facilitator, if necessary. Time constraints for Red Teaming tools are not hard and fast; however, you want to avoid cutting off good discussion, and if there is simply no passion around a planned topic, there is no point in artificially extending the conversation. The facilitators need to set general time limits to ensure the program achieves its goals during the time available for the program. Facilitators can also assign someone from the group to keep time for each tool; this is also a good way to engage team members.

Graphics

This element of presentation is very important. Each Red Team needs to have someone who is facile with online graphics beyond mere PowerPoint skills. Being able to attach short videos or exciting graphics and presenting a professional product is a very important component of successful out-briefs.

Step 5: Present Results

The Red Team should develop the method for presenting the results to the project leader or initiator. Similar to writing a manuscript, a good technique for presenting results is to tell them what you are going to tell them, tell them, and then tell them what you told them. In other words, outline the approach, present the findings, and summarize the recommendations. Box 5.8 presents a typical presentation methodology. In some cases, it is advisable to describe the method that will be used to present the results in detail, to get the boss or project leader to buy-in to the approach before revealing the results. This is particularly true if the results are likely to be met with resistance. If the leader accepts each step of the method, it will be harder for them to dismiss results they do not like. Like everything else associated with Red Teaming, there is no set answer. There are times when setting out the methodology for the presentation will sidetrack or distract from the presentation. Experience, judgement, and rehearsal are the key to determining the best approach.

Explain the Red Team tools that were used well enough so the audience knows this effort was not done in the traditional way but used a reliable, valid, and innovative approach to problem solving. It takes education and practice to become fluent in the use of a tool. The leader or audience to whom the Red Team presents does not have time for fluency. However, it is important they understand the underlying dynamics and rationale for the use of each tool.

The outcomes are more likely to be interpreted as valid, if the audience knows the tools used leveraged anonymity and reflected an overriding perspective of the group. There are many ways to communicate to the audience the nature of the tools, such as graphics, handouts, and testimonials by the Red Team members.

Embrace storytelling as a way to describe alternative futures. Storytelling is an important and effective way to relay complex information in an understandable and memorable way. The kind of stories told during the presentation should challenge conventional thought and are important. Stories should be supported by data or some form of evidence. Even when telling a story about a future event (*pre-mortem analysis*), those imagined events need to be grounded in evidence of current or past action. If the stories told do not resonate and are not believable, then the Red Team will not be credible.

Box 5.8 Typical Presentation Methodology
1. Introduce the Red Team members and provide some background on Red Teaming.
2. Instruct the audience that the Red Team has been asked to use Red Teaming to review the plan/project/question or issue.
3. Use storytelling to convey complex information in an understandable way.
4. Offer the Red Team's recommendations.

> **Box 5.9 Preparing the Presentation**
> 1. Consider assigning roles to some of the team during the rehearsal through which they are designated to listen to the presentation as if they were one of the expected opponents in the room.
> 2. If possible, rehearse with someone from the team that will ultimately hear the presentation. Get their perspective on how the presentation is likely to be received.
> 3. If necessary, change some of the language to soften the blow, but resist changing the actual findings, unless the person with whom the Red Team rehearsed provides new information.
> 4. Red Team your presentation internally to look for flaws.
> 5. Rehearse, rehearse, rehearse.

The Red Team facilitator must constantly monitor the reactions to Red Team feedback among the audience. Sometimes an item that seems fairly mild to the Red Team will anger or upset one of the decision-makers listening to the presentation. In that case, a conscious abandonment of the rehearsed presentation may be necessary to ensure the issue is addressed and satisfied. Conversely, an issue the Red Team thought would be contentious might be accepted immediately, in which case the team should accept the response and not create controversy where there is none. The entire Red Team has the responsibility for reading or sensing the tone of the audience, but is a specific task of the Red Team leader.

The Red Team needs a polished, well-rehearsed presentation that the members have Red Teamed for flaws. Box 5.9 lists some tips on preparing the presentation.

When a new Red Team debuts, it has several things going against it. First, Red Teaming itself may be considered by others to be unproven, a waste of time, and an unnecessary barrier. The object of the Red Team is to challenge the planning or decision-making of the boss or project team so those receiving the presentation are likely to be resistant. The very notion of a team designed to examine "my" work is objectionable to some people, irrespective of the results of the effort. A good example is when accreditors conduct site visits and then out-brief the SON or clinical organization with their findings. It is usually hard to hear about the flaws and weaknesses in the organization. People tend to take the news personally.

Hit a home run. It is not sufficient for a Red Team to make recommendations around the margin. Minor revisions to a plan or project, such as corrections of spelling on slides or to minor misstatements of fact are not why an organization invests in Red Teaming. They do so only because the independent, informed review by a Red Team helps them substantially improve what they are about to do or helps avoid a previously unforeseen pitfall in the future. If the Red Team does not provide either, then the life of Red Teaming in the organization will be limited.

Final Advice

Red Teaming does not fix toxic leaders. If you work for one, do not Red Team! There are some leaders who revel in control and authority. These leaders are certain they are the smartest people in the room. Red Teaming will not convince them otherwise. The best advice to people who find themselves working for leaders who personify these characteristics is to polish up their resume and look for work elsewhere.

Reference

1. George ML, Rowlands D, Price M, Maxey J. The lean six sigma pocket toolbook. New York/London: McGraw-Hill; 2005.

Part II
Cases

Budget Cuts at Green University

6

Issue/Problem Green University is a medium-sized public university. As a result of the ongoing pandemic crisis, the university is in serious financial trouble. The President has asked the deans to cut the budget for the coming academic year and to develop a plan for the fall semester.

Background The School of Nursing (SON) offers a 4-year Bachelors of Science (BSN) degree in nursing. Students are admitted in the freshmen year but begin clinical practice in the junior year. The SON also offers a doctorate of nursing practice with a focus on nurse practitioner programs, a master's degree, and a doctor of philosophy (PhD) in nursing. As part of a multipronged effort to gather as much data as possible to prepare for the fall, the SON dean hires a consultant to facilitate her leadership team through a budget review using Red Teaming methods. The consultant, Jeffre, brings two of his team members to assist with this project. Jeffre and his partners conduct four, 4-hour sessions over 4 weeks with the dean's team. Invited participants include the SON dean, the associate dean for academic affairs, the program directors for the undergraduate, masters, and doctoral programs, and the dean's assistant (who is assisting the team, but is not a full participant).

Solving the Problem

Before engaging the dean's team, Jeffre and his partners spend an hour working directly with the dean to understand the preferred outcomes to tailor the event to her needs. After much discussion, the dean identifies three items she is interested in developing:

1. A set of indicators that will let her know how bad the pandemic is likely to be during the next year.
2. A list of reductions to make immediately and those to delay.
3. An implementation strategy for implementing the reductions.

© The Author(s), under exclusive license to Springer Nature Switzerland AG 2021
L. Neal-Boylan, S. Rotkoff, *Innovative Decision Making in Healthcare*,
https://doi.org/10.1007/978-3-030-72648-5_6

After meeting with the dean, Jeffre and his partners decide to conduct three sessions with the dean's team.

Session One

During the first session, Jeffre introduces the concept of Red Teaming and the methods to be used. He presents the history of Red Teaming and explains the objectives inherent in using Red Teaming methods, such as stirring the imagination and critical thinking about the future, mitigating groupthink, improving listening skills, and making better decisions (Box 6.1). He assures the group members that all the tools and methods used in Red Teaming are aimed at ensuring the best idea wins, instead of the idea with the most powerful advocate.

One of Jeffre's colleagues then explains that group members will engage and communicate in the group using eight techniques (Box 6.2).

Jeffre starts the discussion by asking everyone to *anonymously* forecast what the worst plausible scenario might be for fall enrollment. Jeffre's colleagues distribute note cards and pencils while Jeffre asks everyone to write their own responses on their individual card. Jeffre's partners collect the cards after everyone has had a chance to write a response. (This exercise can be conducted online with each person emailing their answer to the facilitator.) After collecting the cards, Jeffre shares the answers with the group and encourages group discussion. As the discussion ensues, the group focuses on two different possible outcomes:

Box 6.1 Red Team Objectives
- Stir the imagination.
- Think critically about the future.
- Mitigate groupthink.
- Improve listening skills.
- Make better decisions.

Box 6.2 Jeffre's Choices for Red Teaming Techniques
- Anonymous participation.
- Think-write-share.
- Round Robin.
- Open discussion.
- Small groups, including role play.
- Ad Agency.
- Yes, and….
- Best of breed.

1. Reduced freshman enrollment due to national trends, but retention of the majority of sophomores, juniors, and seniors.
2. More people will want to become nurses as a result of the pandemic and, given the financial crisis at the university, the SON will be pressured to take more freshman and additional transfer students into the upper undergraduate cohorts. There will be increased enrollment in the master's degree program. Enrollment of the DNP and PhD students is expected to remain largely the same as before the pandemic.

The group then votes *anonymously* and agrees that the second possible outcome is the most probable. The exercise allows the group to move forward with everyone having had a voice, but with one single and agreed-upon target for the future.

Implementing *think-write-share*, Jeffre then asks everyone to spend some individual time thinking about, and then writing down, internal metrics within their specific areas that might be used as indicators that the second possible outcome was actually happening. Consequently, the dean focuses her thinking on higher level aspects of school operations. The associate dean focuses on curriculum and overarching curricular factors and student needs for support. The BSN program director concentrates on the undergraduate program, and the master's and doctoral program directors concentrate on their specific programs. Jeffre instructs the dean's team to include details they already track (such as transfer admission rate) but might use differently and to come up with a minimum of two items they generally do not track but should consider. Jeffre asks them to propose three factors external to the SON that might impact enrollment and retention in the fall.

Contrary to the first exercise, during this second exercise, responses are shared among the team and are not anonymous. As a result of this discussion, each member of the dean's team develops a dashboard of items they can track that will give them some indication of how enrollment is unfolding. Once they have established items, they will track to ensure their enrollment projections are coming true, they develop the second-order effects of that future state in each of their areas. Box 6.3 captures the primary concerns of each person in coping with their expected future state of increased enrollment. (Box 6.3).

Box 6.3 Issues Associated with Increased Enrollment
- *Dean*: Budget – can it accommodate increased enrollment? Will we have sufficient personnel, space, equipment?
- *Associate Dean*: We will need more resources to provide academic support to increased number of students; will need additional sections to accommodate more students.
- *BSN Program Director*: We will need more clinical placements, more clinical faculty.
- *Master's Program Director and DNP Program Director*: We will need more clinical placements, preceptors, and course sections.
- *Doctoral Program Directors*: We may not have sufficient faculty if BSN and master's programs pull faculty into teaching additional sections in their programs.

Jeffre ends session one by giving the dean's team homework for session two. He asks each member to consider how they will address the issues identified in Box 6.3. Consequently, the dean will review the SON budget to determine how to pay adjunct faculty or faculty overload to teach additional students and consider the space issues inherent in increased enrollment. The associate dean will explore the consequences for the lab and simulation suites, considering the need for additional equipment and supplies, including personal protective equipment. He will also consider the need for additional academic support for increased numbers of students. How will this impact the tutoring and writing centers on campus? The BSN, master's, and DNP program directors will consider the likelihood of clinical placement availability for the current students during the pandemic and the possibility of needing to place additional students. The PhD program has several international students who will not be able to return to campus. Can they continue?

Jeffre asks the dean's team to put their items in three buckets: (1) what is immediately possible to implement, (2) what we will implement only if we must, and (3) what we cannot do under any circumstances. Jeffre asks each member (except the dean's assistant) to send their list to him 24 hours prior to session two. (See Box 6.4 for key points to consider and Box 6.5 for the bucket lists).

Session Two

Before session two begins, Jeffre distributes a document to each team member that includes everyone's ideas without the names of the group members who submitted them. Jeffre asks each person to review the proposed ideas and develop the best compilation reduced to six specific categories:

1. Personnel
   - Adjuncts
   - Additional faculty workload
   - Volunteers
2. Space
   - On campus totally
   - On campus partially

Box 6.4 Key Points to Consider from Session One
- Determined there are two possible outcomes.
- Agreed to focus on the most likely outcome.
- Assessed individual metrics based on each person's area of responsibility within the SON.
- Consideration of consequences of the outcome for each person's area of responsibility.
- Three buckets.

Box 6.5 Bucket Lists

	Immediately possible to implement	Implement only if we must	We cannot do under any circumstances
Dean	Redistribute faculty workload Pay faculty overload Hire more adjuncts Consider reconfiguration of space to accommodate additional course sections Confer with provost and registrar regarding space available across campus Ask for donations of equipment and supplies from community partners and donors	Temporarily halt committee meetings to accommodate the additional faculty workload	Hire new faculty Increase students per classroom or clinical section; we are at our allowable maximum already
Associate dean	Use weekends to hold lab sections and simulation classes to accommodate increased enrollment Meet with writing center and tutoring center to consider options for accommodating increased enrollment	Ask the Office of Advancement and Development to help with donations of PPE and other supplies Ask retired faculty or graduate students to help with academic support and/or tutoring.	Add students to currently enrolled lab and simulation sections since they are already at maximum capacity
BSN program director; Master's program director; DNP program director	Recruit more adjuncts or ask for more time from adjuncts we currently use Explore new options for clinical placements; placements we do not typically use and placements out of state	Increase our use of simulation up to the allowable 50% to provide enough clinical experience to students	We will not be able to get more clinical placements in local hospitals because we are currently at our maximum
PhD program director	Temporarily suspend PhD program for new cohorts Have students who are permitted by their countries to take courses online to do so		We cannot increase online learning to all PhD students because several countries do not allow this for PhD students

- How many students per classroom (for safety)
- Reconfiguring rooms we already have
3. Academic support for students
   - Online only
   - Hire retired faculty or graduate students to provide additional tutoring and support on campus in the SON or ask them to volunteer their time
   - Direct students to the usual resources on campus

4. Lab and simulation
   • Work with current donors to pay for additional needs
   • Petition the provost to pay for additional needs
   • Cut budget elsewhere to pay for additional needs
5. Clinical placements
   • Place only the seniors and NP students
   • Conduct all clinicals virtually
   • Place everyone in clinicals in-person
   • Increase use of simulation
6. PhD international students
   • Defer international students until next semester/next year
   • Conduct classes online
   • Temporarily suspend the program

Each member of the dean's team reviews the compiled list and writes their own recommendations in each of the six categories. After everyone has reviewed the compiled list and built their recommendations in each category, Jeffre conducts an *open discussion* in each area using the *Round Robin* method. As a result, the discussion evolves to further streamline the lists into two main foci: (1) hire or do not hire adjuncts and (2) conduct all classes and clinicals virtually or not.

By the end of session two, the group has established a set of indicators for a dashboard to provide warnings regarding how the future might unfold and has agreed on whether or not to hire adjuncts and whether or not to hold classes and clinicals virtually. (See Box 6.6 for points to consider from session two).

The last task is to develop an implementation strategy. In preparation for session three, Jeffre gives everyone more homework. He breaks the group into two teams of three without the dean in either team. Jeffre tells each team to assign responsibility for each of the following:

1. One person responsible for building an implementation plan around *personnel*.
2. One person responsible for determining how to arrange obtaining sufficient *supplies* in the lab and simulation suites and protecting students and faculty with personal protective equipment in the classrooms and labs.
3. One person responsible for addressing *space* and the international PhD students.

Box 6.6 Key Points to Consider from Session Two
• Review compiled list of six categories.
• Make individual recommendations in each category.
• Open discussion: hire/do not hire adjuncts and all classes/clinicals to be virtual or not.
• Dashboard of warning signs to anticipate the future.

This portion of the session employs *role play* because each person within the group assumes the role of the person responsible for a particular area of responsibility. Each team member is asked to come to session three with their strategy for implementation.

Session Three

Session three is centered on the use of the *Ad Agency* tool (Fig. 6.1) described in Chapter Four. As a reminder, the purpose of this tool is to foster several effective Red Teaming methods simultaneously. First, it puts everyone into a *yes,…and* frame of mind (Chapter 3). Second, it begins with small groups and aggregates to foster creative solutions. Finally, it results in looking at the same problem through a variety of different lenses.

This tool works best when there are three separate but related aspects of the plan being developed or the problem solved, or if there are three different approaches under consideration. Jeffre uses the *Ad Agency* method (Box 6.7) with the two subgroups of the dean's team. The dean is not present. Jeffre instructs the two teams that one person in each subgroup will represent "personnel," another "supplies," and another "space."

Step 1: Jeffre directs that each team member MUST design a smart approach to reducing expenditures in their assigned area (personnel, supplies, or space). They cannot debate the wisdom of doing so, they have been directed to do so and must

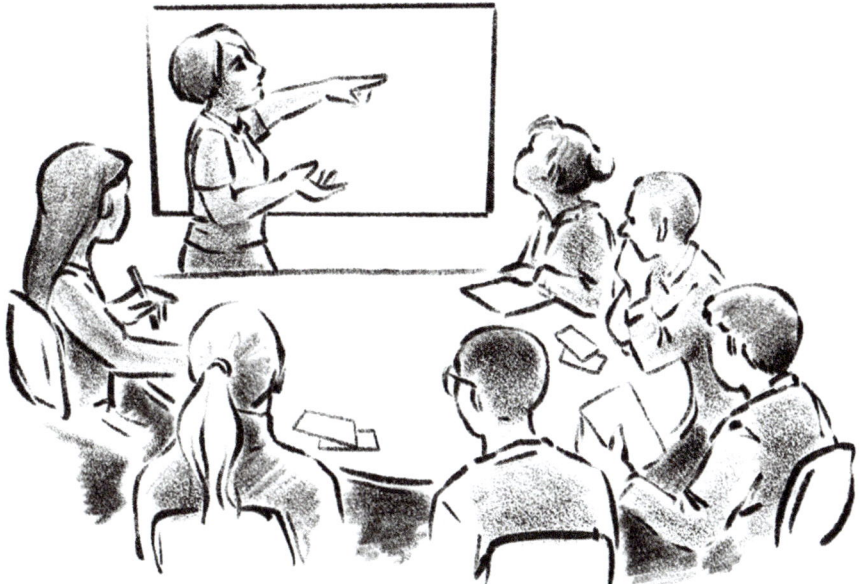

Fig. 6.1 Ad Agency (Drawings provided by Tara J. Neal @TaraNealArts)

Box 6.7 Summary of Application of the *Ad Agency* Strategy in the SON at Green University

(a) Each team member designs a smart approach to reducing expenditures in their assigned area (personnel, supplies, or space).

(b) Each person designs their approach independent of the other team members.

(c) The three-person team comes together. The representative (advocate) for personnel is the client and presents his/her ideas to the other two team members.

(d) The advocate leaves the room while the other two team members discuss the advocate's proposal.

(e) The advocate or client returns to the team to listen to feedback from the other two team members.

(f) This process (c and d) are repeated for the advocates of supplies and space.

(g) New teams are formed. The two advocates for personnel meet. The two advocates for supplies meet. The two advocates for space meet.

(h) Each of these new teams then presents their proposal to the entire group including the dean.

(i) The dean decides on the final strategy based on the proposals presented.

(j) The dean assigns tasks to each team member to implement the final strategy.

design the best way to implement the approach to save the most money with the least impact on revenue generation and quality of education.

Step 2: Each person in each team works to design their approach independently without consultation of the other team members.

Step 3: Once each person has designed their plan, they sit in a small circle with the other two team members. The advocate for a plan concerning personnel (option one) speaks first. The other two members who serve as the *Ad Agency* listen and take notes. After the team member presenting option one has finished their presentation, they walk away and give the "Ad Agency" time to talk about the option one proposal.

Step 4: The *Ad Agency* must find ways to improve instead of dismiss the option one proposal. Like an advertising agency, they cannot tell the client he/she is wrong or ignorant; instead, they must build on and improve the client's ideas. They consult with each other first without the client present so they can speak openly about the ideas and consider how to improve them.

Step 5: The client (the team member who presented option one) returns to the *Ad Agency* and listens to the team's feedback on how to improve the idea. The client asks questions to understand their feedback and takes notes.

Steps 3–5 are then repeated. The team members representing supplies present their ideas to the other two members of their team. The team members representing space then present their ideas to the other two members of their team. The team members advocating for their area play the role of client in these scenarios.

The teams now separate into the committee members who represented each option. The two committee members representing personnel come together and build a list of the best ideas to save money with the least impact. The committee members representing supplies and the team members representing space do the same thing. Each team builds a *best of breed* list to present to the dean and the entire group (See Box 6.8 for Key Points to consider for sessions three and four and Box 6.9 for Best of Breed results).

Box 6.8 Key Points to Consider from Sessions Three and Four
- Design smart approaches for reducing expenditures for personnel, supplies, and space.
- Best of breed list.

Box 6.9 Best of Breed in This Case

Option one (personnel): Decrease or stop all committee work for the time being and add courses to full-time faculty workload, thereby saving money on adjuncts. Incentivize faculty to take on more courses or sections by considering bonuses or a significantly reduced credit load during a future semester. Hire only as many adjuncts as we absolutely need. Recruit volunteers to provide additional academic support during this time.

Option two (supplies): Require students to bring and wear their own masks. Provide hand sanitizer, face shields, and gloves and have each student store these in a paper bag with their name on it in a designated locker to use each time they come to the lab. Make some disposable items reusable.

Option three (space): Check temperatures of all students, faculty, and staff at the door of the building. Allow only four, instead of eight students in the lab at one time and have them sit using social distancing guidelines. Each student will work alone with each lab mannequin or at each exam table to practice and demonstrate skills. The other four students in the lab class attend on a different day (possibly weekends) or time and do the same thing. During the pandemic, give all students the option of attending theory classes online or on campus. Convert the cafeteria (since it is not in use during the pandemic) to a lab to fit more students. Use simulation to maximum allowable amount of 50% for clinical experiences. Use virtual clinical experiences whenever possible to augment in-person experiences. Store conference room furniture to create more space for teaching students.

International students: Allow those who can participate online to do so and defer admissions or continuing of the program for those students who are not permitted by their countries to take classes online.

This process (including the final briefing to the entire dean's team and the dean) takes the entire session. At the end of the session, the dean hands out tasks to the dean's team to ensure the dashboard is in place, and that the implementation strategy can be affected.

The *Ad Agency* strategy enabled the dean to hear the voices of her senior staff, the people who will ultimately need to implement the final strategy. This is not the end of the story, however. The dean will then explain to the faculty her decision and the Red Team process she used to reach that decision. Faculty will have the opportunity to weigh in on the decision but can be reassured that a considered, deliberative process was used to reach the decision. It is likely that any objections raised by the faculty will have already been considered through this Red Team process.

Critical Thinking Questions

1. Why was it preferable in this case to break this issue up into several work sessions?
2. What were the advantages to using Red Team methods to resolve the issue?
3. How can the dean be confident that everyone in her leadership team had an opportunity to be heard?

Horizontal Violence in Pink Hospital

7

Problem/Issue The nursing literature is replete with descriptions of horizontal violence among nurses in clinical settings [1]. This has been known to contribute to new nurse burnout and attrition [2–4]. This case describes a hypothetical case of horizontal violence and bullying and how the nurse manager might use Red Team methods to help resolve the problem. The case takes place in a hospital but could be applicable to other clinical and academic settings.

Background Corinne is a new nurse on a medical-surgical floor at a small community hospital. She just graduated from a BSN program and is excited about her first job. She was a good but not stellar student and found nursing school intense and demanding. She struggled in her theory classes, but did well in her clinical placements. She feels anxious but thinks she has been well prepared to begin her new role.

Corinne has a 2-week full-time orientation during which she learns the hospital's policies and procedures and gets a comprehensive tour. She wanted to work in a hospital that provided a new nurse residency program, but she lives with her parents in this small town and does not want to move for a few more years. Corinne enjoys meeting other new nurses during the orientation and is excited when she is told it is time to move to the unit.

Corinne is assigned to Kendall, a nurse who has worked in this hospital for 30 years and on the unit for 20 of those years. Kendall greets Corinne on her first day on the unit. Corinne is 10 minutes late to her shift because her bus was late. Kendall is dressed in clean permanent press scrubs and is wearing a lab coat and her hospital identification badge. Corinne has dumped her bag and coat in the break room and rushes to meet Kendall at the nurse's station. Kendall's first impression of Corinne is that she is late and unkempt in appearance. Over the years, Kendall has oriented countless new nurses to the unit. With few exceptions, she has found new graduate nurses to be slovenly, unprofessional, and lacking in knowledge about the basics needed to provide care independently. Kendall prides herself on having weeded out the weaker nurses and trained the others to be excellent nurses who still work in her

L. Neal-Boylan, S. Rotkoff, *Innovative Decision Making in Healthcare*,
https://doi.org/10.1007/978-3-030-72648-5_7

unit. From Kendall's perspective, Corinne has failed her first test. Kendall gives Corinne a stern warning to always be on time with no excuses and to look and act in a professional manner. She tells Corinne to cut her nails, shed the nail polish, and get rid of the blue tints in her hair and the ring in her nose. She tells Corinne "that may have been acceptable in school but this is the real world honey." Corinne nods her head in agreement and follows Kendall the rest of the day trying to do her best to be professional. Later, Corinne is able to talk to some other nurses from her orientation who are experiencing the same type of treatment from the senior staff on their units. Kendall tells her experienced colleagues that she has had it with these new graduates and might consider retirement.

Solving the Problem

After several weeks, Corinne is sitting in the break room crying because Kendall has just scolded her again. Norah, the unit manager sees her when she goes in to get her lunch out of the refrigerator. Corinne tries to hide her tears and look professional, but Norah sits down beside her and asks what is going on. Corinne, who is contemplating quitting, decides she has nothing to lose and confides in Norah. Corinne explains that she feels bullied by Kendall and recently some of the other more experienced nurses have also been unkind to her. Corinne says she has spoken to her peers on other units and they are having similar experiences.

Norah thanks Corinne for disclosing this and returns to her office to consider the matter. Norah is aware that new nurses have always had to go through a rite of passage in their first jobs. However, a recent conference Norah attended included a seminar that explained "horizontal violence" and that this form of bullying was increasing. Norah decides to meet with Corinne and the other newly or recently hired nurses on her unit in an informal focus group. She asks them to discuss their experiences on the unit without mentioning horizontal violence or bullying. To her surprise, none of the nurses, including Corinne, say anything negative about their experiences. Norah holds a similar informal focus group with the more experienced/older nurses on the unit and asks them how they think the newer nurses are doing. This group is more vocal; the session gets out of control because the nurses are talking over one another to complain about the newer nurses.

Norah recognizes that she needs some help and consults the hospital's chief nurse. The chief nurse, Bonnie, understands that this might be a hospital-wide problem, so she convenes groups consisting of young nurses and experienced nurses (the stakeholders) from across the hospital. She conducts these meetings during all three shifts so everyone has a chance to participate. Participation is largely voluntary, but she is sure to include Corinne and Kendall as well as some carefully chosen newly hired and experienced nurses Bonnie knows are likely to have concerns.

Bonnie employs Red Team methods to work with the groups (Box 7.1).

Box 7.1 Red Team methods Used in this Case
- Anonymous feedback.
- 4 ways of seeing.
- Think-write-share.
- 1–2–4–all.
- Second chance meeting.

Box 7.2 Results of 4 Ways of Seeing Exercise

Group X (experienced nurses) sees their own roles in relation to the new nurses (Group Y):

Orienting the new nurses to the unit and the unit's formal and informal policies.

Group X sees the roles of the new nurses (Group Y):

To closely observe how things are done, learn the unit and hospital policies, research what they do not know by using online resources or their books from school, help all the staff to care for the patients, and care for their own patients. Group X members comment that the new nurses have graduated from nursing programs and should know what they are doing at a novice level and not have to bother the experienced nurses (Group X) so much.

Group Y (new nurses) see their own roles as:

Applying what they have learned in school to the real world, learning what they need to know to be good nurses, caring safely for patients.

Group Y sees the roles of Group X in relation to the new nurses as:

Mentoring new nurses to learn how to be good nurses to and to work on the unit; being a resource to the new nurses as they learn; teaching and nurturing the new nurses while they adapt to their new roles and the unit.

First, she requests anonymous feedback by asking the experienced nurses to describe what they see as their role on their units. She also asks them to anonymously list what they think the role and behavior should be of the new nurses. (Recall the description of the *4 ways of seeing* tool in Chapter Three.) Bonnie is aiming to try to get group X (experienced nurses) to see their roles as they relate to the new nurses and how they see the roles of the new nurses (group Y). She meets with groups of new nurses and asks them to do the converse (how they see their own roles in relation to the experienced nurses and how they see the roles of the experienced nurses). Box 7.2 lists the results of this *4 ways of seeing* exercise.

Bonnie learns a lot from this exercise, especially that the experienced nurses and new nurses have very different perspectives of their roles in relation to each other. She discusses the findings with her leadership team and decides the next step is to combine the experienced and new nurses to address the areas of conflict. Bonnie begins each meeting by reporting on the results of the *4 ways of seeing* and the focus groups.

Bonnie enlists Norah to help her conduct the *think-write-share* (T-W-S) and *1-2-4-all* exercises on all three shifts. Bonnie and Norah pair an experienced nurse with a new nurse in each of the groups that attend these mandatory meetings. Bonnie asks each person to *think* about the issue of conflict between experienced nurses and new nurses. After giving everyone several minutes to think, she asks each person to *write* down what they think should be done to resolve the conflicts. Then, each person *shares* their ideas with their partner.

Norah facilitates a general large group discussion by asking each pair to share their ideas with the larger group. Once this has been done and the ideas have been listed on a white board, she groups two pairs together into groups of four. Each team of four (two experienced nurses and two new nurses) discuss potential solutions to the conflicts and determine who will be their team's spokesperson. Bonnie then directs each spokesperson to rotate to another group and share the ideas from their own team. Each group to whom the spokesperson rotates listens to the ideas and adds to them using the *Yes, and...* method.

Once each spokesperson has rotated to each of the other groups, they bring the ideas they have accumulated back "home" to their own team. The team then refines their ideas based on the feedback the spokesperson received. Finally, Bonnie asks each spokesperson to report out to the large group. Box 7.3 lists the results of these Red Team methods.

Bonnie reminds everyone that all nurses work as a team and should not work against each other. She directs that the ideas in Box 7.2 be put in writing and that

---

Box 7.3 Results of the *T-W-S, 1-2-4-all* and *Yes, and...* Methods
Experienced nurses:

- Orient new nurses to the unit.
- Orient new nurses to the policies and procedures of the unit.
- Serve as resources for information.
- Provide a support system for new nurses.

New nurses:

- Come to work on time and dress and act professionally.
- Come to work prepared to take care of the types of patients we care for in our unit, i.e., review what you learned in school, read the journals, and subscribe to free or low-cost online continuing education programs.
- Unless it is an emergency, try to find the answer to your question before seeking information from the experienced nurses who are busy caring for their own patients.
- Start each day receptive to learning.

everyone make an effort to abide by them. She tells the nurses that she plans to reconvene the groups in 6 months to assess how things are going. Bonnie meets with Norah and the rest of her leadership team and informs them of the results of the meetings. She asks them to assist the nurses on their units to abide by the ideas they developed. (See Box 7.4 for key considerations in this case).

Six Months Later

Bonnie and Norah reconvene the groups of nurses, meeting with each shift. They use the *second chance meeting* (Chap. 3) approach to review the last 6 months. Bonnie and Norah co-facilitate a discussion to determine whether nurses were able to comply with the strictures listed in Box-7.3. As a result of this discussion, each shift suggests tweaks to the original plan. The new nurses verbalize that they are feeling more confident in their roles and that the experienced nurses have been less aggressive and more supportive. However, as a group they still perceive some subliminal hostility. They also protest that they do not have time to pursue continuing education or read journals. Most are working 12-hour shifts and have their own families. They state that as much as they love nursing, they view it as a job not their entire life.

The experienced nurses report that the new nurses have improved in both their competence and willingness to "do their homework" before approaching the experienced nurses with every question. As a group, they feel more inclined to help and support the new nurses. Contrary to the new nurses, the experienced nurses believe nursing is a calling, not a job and while they do not neglect their families, they think nursing goes beyond the shift and is a way of life.

Second chance meeting helps Bonnie and Norah understand that there are fundamental differences between the two groups. These differences might never change, but with continued intentional effort, both groups can constitute a solid working team whose primary purpose is providing high quality care to patients.

Critical Thinking Questions

1. Given tensions between new and experienced nurses, would it be preferable to use Red Team methods that insured anonymity rather than open discussion?
2. Could the Red Team methods described in this case be used on the unit level rather than the hospital level?
3. Do the issues of horizontal violence and bullying go beyond communication between new and experienced nurses? What role does hospital culture play? How does nursing education in schools of nursing play a role? Is the nursing profession as a whole successfully dealing with this issue on a larger scale?

References

1. Bloom EM. Horizontal violence among nurses: experiences, responses, and job performance. Nurs Forum. 2019;54:77–83. https://doi.org/10.1111/nuf.12300.
2. Guo Y, Luo Y, Lam L, Cross W, Plummer V, Zhang J. Burnout and its association with resilience in nurses: a cross-sectional study. J Clin Nurs. 2017; https://doi.org/10.1111/jocn.13952.
3. Rawal CN, Pardeshi SA. Job stress causes attrition among nurses in public and private hospitals. IOSR J Nurs Health Sci. 2014; https://doi.org/10.9790/1959-03224247.
4. Rushton CH, Batcheller J, Schroeder K, Donohue P. Burnout and resilience among nurses practicing in high-intensity settings. Am J Crit Care. 2017;24(5):412–20.

Strategic Planning at Yellow Institute

8

Problem/Issue

The SON at Yellow Institute has moved from a department to a school and needs a new strategic plan.

Background

Yellow Institute is a small private college located in a rural setting. For several years, the Institute had a department of nursing, but 3 years ago, the Board of Trustees approved the transition of the department to a school of nursing (SON). The provost initially appointed the department chair as the interim dean, but a successful search was conducted and the inaugural dean is now in place.

The new dean is leading ten tenured or tenure track faculty, nine teaching and clinical faculty, and two administrative staff. The dean has determined that it is time to begin developing a new strategic plan for the SON. The department of nursing had a strategic plan but, as an independent school, the organizational structure and priorities have changed.

The SON dean proposes asking one of the business faculty who specializes in strategic planning to assist in this work. She requests the provost provide a stipend for the business faculty with a reduced teaching load for the upcoming academic year. This will make the business faculty more available to the SON.

Solving the Problem Kevin is the business faculty who has agreed to work with the SON. Kevin arranges three meetings: One with the dean and associate dean, another with the program directors, and one with the faculty. Following these meetings, everyone will meet in a 2-day retreat.

The meeting with the dean is critical to helping Kevin better understand her priorities and how Red Team capabilities can help her reach her desired outcomes. The dean decides a 2-day retreat will allow the faculty and staff to focus on strategic planning without other distractions. The retreat is scheduled for the period

© The Author(s), under exclusive license to Springer Nature Switzerland AG 2021
L. Neal-Boylan, S. Rotkoff, *Innovative Decision Making in Healthcare*,
https://doi.org/10.1007/978-3-030-72648-5_8

following the December holidays prior to the beginning of spring semester. The dean's objectives for the retreat include the following:

1. Assist the SON faculty to take the prior strategic plan including the institution's nine Strategic Pillars or overarching goals, and re-prioritize the strategic priorities (SP) the department of nursing had developed in alignment with the pillars. The SON's strategic plan should be in alignment with the institute's plan so there is no intention to change or delete any of the pillars.
2. Help the faculty and staff determine which activities they are currently doing that they can stop doing.
3. Set the stage to begin work on the SON's new or revised strategic priorities and create new action steps to align with each Strategic Pillar.

Kevin meets with the associate dean to understand his strategic priorities from a curriculum perspective. He also meets with the program directors for the baccalaureate, doctor of nursing practice (DNP), and PhD programs. He assists the program directors to brainstorm to envision potential futures for the SON. Kevin records their anonymous ideas so he can refer to them later in the process.

During the following month, the dean, the associate dean, and Kevin exchange several emails and phone calls designed to ensure a quality retreat that will meet the needs of the SON.

Several days prior to the first day of the retreat, Kevin sends a message to the SON administrators and faculty. He attaches the department of nursing strategic plan and asks everyone to think about the priorities the SON should pursue over the next 3 years. He asks everyone to thoughtfully consider changes in the profession, the needs of the communities of interest (local community including agencies that employ nursing graduates, students, faculty, and staff) and projected changes in healthcare.

The current strategic plan includes the nine institutional pillars, the department of nursing strategic priorities (three strategic priorities are listed under each pillar), and several action steps for each SP (Box 8.1). To prepare for the retreat, Kevin asks participants to individually and anonymously rank the current SPs within each pillar based on three criteria:

1. Does this SP still apply now that the department of nursing is a school?
2. How urgent is this SP?
3. How easily could the SPs within each pillar be implemented?

Box 8.1 Sample Pillar with Strategic Priorities and Action Steps
I. Pillar: Enhance interdisciplinary education.
   (a) Strategic priority (SP): Increase exposure of nursing students in all degree programs to students in other health related disciplines.

Action step:
1. Develop a formal committee with faculty from across the institute to discuss interdisciplinary courses and activities.
2. Send interested nursing faculty to continuing education programs to learn more about interprofessional education.
3. Obtain grant funding to foster interdisciplinary activities and course development.

Box 8.2 Red Team Strategies for This Case
- Dot voting.
- Ad Agency.
- Round Robin.
- Best of breed.

Participants are asked to individually rank the SPs on a scale of 1–10 with 10 being most important. Kevin asks participants to also rank the SPs on a scale of 1–10 with 10 being hardest to implement. Participants are given thresholds they cannot exceed in terms of urgency and difficulty – i.e., they can only give out three 9 s and 10s and are forced to give out at least four 5s and below. (see *Forced Distribution* – Chap. 3) Kevin requires that each participant list their role (dean, program director, faculty, etc.) on their responses before submitting the responses.

Once the participants have individually completed the ranking based on each criterion, they send their work to Kevin who compiles the feedback. In doing so, Kevin separates the responses of the faculty and program directors from those of the dean and associate dean. Kevin develops a plan for the retreat with the approval of the dean (Box 8.2).

Retreat Day 1

On the first day of the retreat after everyone has a chance to greet one another and grab their morning coffee, Kevin presents the data from the prioritization exercise. There are glaring discrepancies between the responses of the dean and associate dean in comparison to the program directors and faculty. It is clear they do not share the same perceptions of the urgency of each strategic priority nor the ease with which the action steps can be implemented.

Kevin engages the entire group (dean, associate dean, program directors, and faculty) in a *dot voting* exercise (Chap. 3). This exercise will bring forward the critical issues to determine those that require initial discussion.

Box 8.3 Use of *Ad Agency* Tool in This Case
1. There are 21 faculty and staff. They are divided into seven groups of three.
2. Each of the three people in the group represents one strategic priority within pillar #1. For example, Tara represents strategic priority #1, Garrett represents strategic priority #2, and Kyle represents #3. (If there are more than three strategic priorities within the pillar, the faculty and staff can be divided differently so there are four or five people per group with one person representing each priority within the pillar).
3. Because there are nine pillars, the *Ad Agency* exercise is repeated for each pillar.
4. During this exercise, some groups create new strategic priorities within Pillar 1.

Kevin then divides the faculty, including the program directors and associate dean (but not the dean), into seven groups of three (with one of each of the three in a group representing one of the three strategic priorities in pillar one). Kevin explains the use of the Red Team tool *Ad Agency* (Chap. 4). Before the exercise begins, the dean describes a few non-negotiables and her rationale. (Box 8.3 describes how the *Ad Agency* tool is applied in this case).

During the morning session, three pillars are completed. Before lunch, Kevin reconvenes everyone into one large group. He asks the advocates from within each group (Pillar One, Pillar Two, and Pillar Three) to make their cases for each of the strategic priorities. For example, Tara from group A makes her case for SP #1 being the most important priority in Pillar One. Her counterparts from the other small groups of three, state their cases about SP #1. After each of the representatives of SP #1 have made their case, the dean asks penetrating questions to clarify their choices and better understand why SP #1 might or might not be easy to implement.

Then, Garrett states his case for SP #2 as a strategic priority. His counterparts from the other groups do the same. The dean again asks questions. Finally, Kyle and his counterparts state their cases for SP #3 and the dean plays her part.

After everyone has been heard, Kevin asks everyone to vote individually and anonymously on the SP they consider to be of highest priority within Pillar One. He asks everyone to consider the effort required to implement and sustain the priority they have chosen. He facilitates a conversation among all faculty and staff (while the dean observes). He utilizes the *Round Robin* technique to ensure no one speaks twice until everyone gets a chance to speak once. He uses a white board to record the ideas that come out of this discussion. Finally, Kevin asks everyone to use an index card to individually and anonymously record which SP they now consider the most urgent *and* possible to implement and sustain (*Best of Breed*, Fig. 8.1).

This same process is conducted for Pillars Two and Three. (See Box 8.4 for Key Points to Consider).

Fig. 8.1 Best of breed

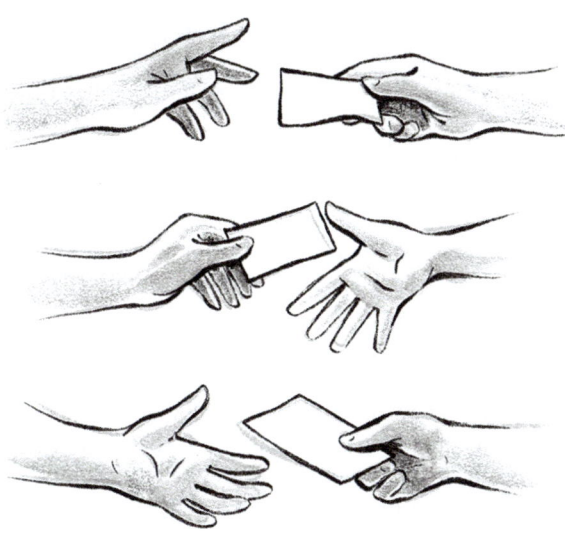

After lunch, the next three pillars are discussed and analyzed using the same process.

Retreat Day 2

The final three pillars are analyzed and reviewed using the same process used during day one of the retreat. The work thus far results in reprioritization within each pillar and new and reordered strategic priorities within each pillar. Some strategic priorities have been discarded, others revised and others created. While this is a great outcome, it is clear there is also a need to identify what the SON should stop doing. This work will be conducted during an extended faculty/staff meeting in 2 weeks' time.

Kevin gives everyone homework to prepare for the next half-day session. He asks that each participant send him their list of which activities the SON should stop doing. The list should include activities both within and outside their control.

Faculty/Staff Meeting Session

Kevin begins the session by sharing his compiled list of the aggregate responses. He breaks the faculty and program directors into groups and uses a *best of breed* approach (Chap. 3).

The dean and the associate dean form their own group and develop their list of what to stop doing. The associate dean and the dean comprise one group, the faculty and staff another group, and the program directors the third group. The groups come back together and share their lists of activities the SON should stop doing. Kevin leads the large group through *weighted anonymous feedback* (using either *dot voting* or *5 will get you 25* both of which weigh issues anonymously (Chap. 3) identifying several items that had the agreement of all three groups.

The dean now has a better understanding of the concerns and perspectives of her staff as a consequence of the process; she shares her rationale from a very different perspective. She explains why she believes some of the things the team wants to stop doing are essential to her as she communicates with the school president, donors, and others. She also yields on things that are more burdensome on her staff than she realized.

Kevin then asks everyone to submit anonymous index cards noting what regarding the newly developed SPs makes them (1) most excited and (2) most concerned. While everyone takes a break, Kevin reviews the feedback and finds the results mostly positive. He repeats this exercise for each pillar.

As a result of this session and the day-and-a-half retreat, the SON has new SPs for each of the nine pillars. The SPs have been reordered or recreated according to urgency and ease of implementation and sustainability. Later, the dean, associate dean, and program directors place the faculty and staff in committees for each pillar. They select who will be in each committee based on the expertise they bring to the specific pillar and how the SPs within the pillar might impact or be impacted by that person. At the next faculty/staff meeting, the dean explains how she chose each committee and has everyone gather in their assigned groups. She charges each committee with working during the spring semester on their particular pillar of the strategic plan. Each group will work to develop new action steps to align with each of the new SPs.

Strategic planning is vitally important to organizations. However, strategic plans can only be useful and realistic if everyone has a voice in the future goals and priorities of the organization. If people do not have a voice, they are less likely to make the effort to implement the plan and are less likely to rejoice when goals are accomplished. This case described how everyone, including staff, had a voice without pursuing priorities that are non-negotiable based on the university's expectations of the dean. In the end, the dean makes the final decisions, but the Red Teaming process ensures everyone has a voice.

Critical Thinking Questions

1. Why might Red Team approaches to strategic planning be more effective than your current method?
2. Do you expect the SON administration to have different perspectives from the faculty and staff?
3. What are the likely consequences if administration assumes most of the responsibility for strategic planning?

Who Is in Charge at Orange School of Nursing

9

Problem/Issue Orange School of Nursing (SON) resides within a college of health sciences (CoHS) in a large public university. The dean of the CoHS consistently overrules decisions made by the SON dean.

Background After a difficult struggle 3 years ago, the Department of Nursing (DON) became a SON. The faculty, along with its union, fought long and hard to demonstrate why the DON should become an SON. One of the biggest antagonists to the proposal was the CoHS dean. She had recently been hired and was enjoying having several departments under her direction. The CoHS dean is a health professional but not a nurse. During the intervening 10 years since the DON became an SON, the CoHS dean has been working closely with the former DON chair in the position of SON dean. The CoHS dean appointed the SON dean with the approval of the provost. The faculty were not involved in the selection of the dean. With the advent of a new provost 3 years ago, the SON was able to win approval for its first official inaugural dean to be selected via the standard selection process involving SON faculty and staff. The search for a new dean began last year and this past summer, the inaugural dean was hired. The selection went through a multilayered process, but faculty and staff played a key role in her selection.

During the interview process, the CoHS dean assured the incoming SON dean that she will have the final decision-making capability for all SON decisions, especially those involving budget and personnel, including hiring and firing. In fact, the posted dean position description confirms this. However, as the academic year wears on, the new SON dean is finding that the CoHS dean insists on weighing in on every decision and in having the last word. Furthermore, the CoHS dean sets up barriers to the SON dean communicating directly with the provost. The SON faculty and staff are aware of the problem. Some of the CoHS dean's staff have also expressed concern with the current arrangement but have done so with SON individuals privately and confidentially. It appears that there will be some support among the CoHS staff to support change.

L. Neal-Boylan, S. Rotkoff, *Innovative Decision Making in Healthcare*,
https://doi.org/10.1007/978-3-030-72648-5_9

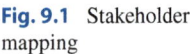 **Fig. 9.1** Stakeholder mapping

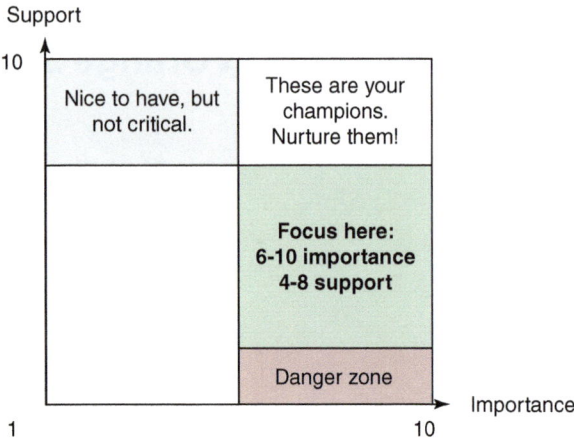

Solving the Problem The SON dean realizes that neither Red Teaming nor any other technique of which she is aware can fix toxic leadership. She recognizes that Red Teaming can only work on what is within one's control. The current organizational structure works for the CoHS dean and she has no reason to alter it. Consequently, solving the problem in this case must focus on how the SON and the SON dean move forward given the current culture.

The SON dean recognizes there is considerable resentment among the SON faculty and staff regarding the current organizational structure of having the CoHS dean approve of or veto every SON decision. Also, faculty and staff have expressed that they feel the SON has stagnated because of the current structure. They hired this dean because she has demonstrated an inclination to be futuristic and innovative and they want to be able to take advantage of that. The SON dean decides the best way to proceed is to help the SON faculty and staff move forward within the structure which means changing the culture in the SON.

The first challenge is to determine who in the SON might be in the best positions to do things differently. Box 9.1 lists the Red Team tools to be used to address this problem. The SON dean, familiar with Red Teaming employs two tools in tandem to better understand the playing field. They are *stakeholder mapping* and *4 ways of seeing*. Recall the illustration from Chap. 4 reprinted below as Fig. 9.1.

Box 9.1 Red Team Tools Used to Solve This Case
- Stakeholder mapping.
- 4 ways of seeing.
- Think-write-share (T-W-S).
- 1-2-4-all.
- Yes, and….
- TRIZ.

Step 1: Before the SON dean meets with all SON faculty and staff, she considers who are the "stakeholders" based on how critical they are to changing the culture in the SON. There may be stakeholders whom the change will affect, but they will have little influence over implementation, and there may be stakeholders without whom new ideas cannot be implemented. At this stage, the SON dean defers assessing whether she thinks each stakeholder may be supportive or opposed to the idea. The only question is how necessary each one is to idea implementation. The SON dean ranks (Box 9.2) those who are very necessary to changing the culture with a "10"; those unnecessary to the implementation of a new culture are ranked at 1, with gradations in between (1–10).

It is important to note that the CoHS dean is not included on either list because while she is very important to any change in culture, she will not be supportive. That is why the SON must change its way of doing things rather than trying to change how the CoHS dean sees herself or her relationship with the SON. Also of note, is the absence of the SON faculty on either list. While they are vitally important to culture change within the SON, the culture change in this case has to do with decisions made within the SON and how they are approved and moved forward despite the barrier of the CoHS dean. Almost all SON decisions require the approval of the faculty. This case pertains to what happens after faculty have approved SON decisions and made their recommendations to the SON dean. The SON dean is then tasked with obtaining CoHS approval and guiding implementation.

Step 2: The SON dean then holds a meeting with all SON faculty and staff in attendance. Without sharing her ranked list, she presents the issue and asks each person to use the *think-write-share* (T-W-S) technique (Chap. 3) to write down who they think will be critical to the process of a change in culture. She asks them to rank them on a scale of 1–10. She then asks them to similarly rank the level of support they associate with each of the stakeholders they identified as critical to the change. The SON faculty and staff build their own version of the list that the SON dean had built individually (Box 9.3).

Based on the stakeholder analysis, the SON dean is confident that everyone on her team is committed to improving the relationship with the CoHS. The key to

Box 9.2 Dean's Ranking in Order of Those Necessary to Changing How the SON Acquires CoHS Approval for SON Decisions

People	Level of importance	Level of support
SON dean	10	10
Chair of SON	10	10
Associate chair of SON	9	10
SON program directors	10	9
SON dean's assistant/office manager	7	9
CoHS associate dean	9	4

Box 9.3 Faculty and Staff Ranking of the Most Important and Most Supportive Stakeholders

People	Level of importance	Level of support
SON dean	10	10
Chair of SON	10	10
Associate chair of SON	9	10
SON program directors	10	10
SON dean's assistant/office manager	0	9
CoHS associate dean	9	3

doing so is developing the associate dean of the CoHS (ADCoHS) as a stronger advocate on behalf of the SON. The ADCoHS is in the position to influence the CoHS dean and is open to supporting the SON. The critical issue is how to best support the ADCoHS in her support of the SON. This requires a better understanding of the perspectives of both organizations; based on this insight the SON dean decides to conduct a *4 ways of seeing* to make the perspectives of the SON and the CoHS more obvious to the entire team.

The 4 ways of seeing she chooses are as follows:

- How does the SON see itself (how X sees X)?
- How does the SON see the CoHS (how X sees Y)?
- How does the CoHS see itself (how Y sees Y)?
- How does the CoHS see the SON (how Y sees X)?

For this effort, she asks the ADCoHs to bring in some of her staff to the Red Team process to represent the perspectives of the CoHS. The results of this effort are listed in Boxes 9.4, 9.5, 9.6, and 9.7.

Box 9.4 How the SON Sees Itself
- We are an accredited school of nursing and our dean should have rights and responsibilities equivalent to the other deans on campus.
- We are the primary revenue source for the CoHS; as such, we should have a greater voice over our own budget and priorities.
- We are a profession that while part of healthcare, is fundamentally different in many ways from the other departments within the CoHS.
- Our priorities need to be nursing centric and unconstrained by the needs or perspective of the CoHS.

Box 9.5 How the SON Sees the CoHS
- The CoHS dean has reserved all power to her office. While we now have our inaugural dean, we are still structured more like a department than a school. Our dean has no power or authority.
- We have to go through the CoHS associate dean for anything pertaining to academic affairs regardless of whether our dean has approved our decisions.
- We should be able to make our own decisions and not have to go through the CoHS associate dean.
- The role of the CoHS associate dean should be that of consultant, if and when we need her input or advice.

Box 9.6 How the CoHS Sees Itself
- The CoHS must approve all academic initiatives and curricula across the CoHS.
- All policies of all departments within the CoHS must adhere to the policies of the CoHS.
- The CoHS dean has been at the school a long time, understands the politics of the school, has a longstanding relationship with the President of the school, and has the charter to supervise all of the schools inside the CoHS.

Box 9.7 How the CoHS Sees the SON
- The SON is a valuable source of revenue to the school.
- The SON is a newly independent school with a new dean.
- The SON is a non-team player, focused only on the needs of the SON, to the exclusion of the needs of the CoHS or the school in general.
- The SON is too focused on establishing authority and independence from the CoHS.

Based on this frank, informed (because of the participation of the ADCoHS) *4 ways of seeing*, it is clear that the SON needs to work hard to establish new means of communication and interact more effectively with the CoHS. To better understand why the communication is so poor, the SON dean decides to conduct a TRIZ (Chap. 4). The object of the TRIZ is to design the worst possible relationship between the SON and the CoHS.

After breaking into groups and asking each group to design the worst possible policies and approaches to ensure a terrible relationship between the SON and the

CoHS, the group discovers that some of those things that created friction in the exercise are already present. For example:

- Because the CoHS has other priorities, it frequently is slow to approve those requests for policy changes that the SON sends forward. This creates a vicious cycle in which the SON is reluctant to seek approval from the CoHS because they are slow to approve and the CoHS is slow to approve because the SON tries to sidestep them whenever possible.
- Also, the SON in keeping with being an accredited SON, has changed its letter-head in a way to identify itself outside the umbrella of the CoHS. While inno-cently done, seen through the eyes of the CoHS, it seems like another effort to separate the SON from the CoHS.
- Because the SON perspective is different from that of the CoHS, the SON dean has publicly disagreed with the CoHS dean in university meetings – also rein-forcing the perception of the lack of team play.

As a result of TRIZ, the SON dean recognizes that the situations described above are happening right now. The SON dean uses *T-W-S* with her faculty and staff to develop some remedies (Box 9.8).

During the course of this exercise, the SON dean has to quell the resentment of SON faculty and staff for the inability to run as an autonomous school and reinforce the need to work within the current organizational structure. She emphasizes that the SON can, over time, gain recognition for making sound and rational decisions in collaboration with the CoHS and with the approval of the CoHS dean. She hopes this will eventually lead to greater autonomy. (Box 9.9 includes key points to con-sider at this point in the case).

Box 9.8 Proposed Remedies

SON dean	The SON dean will propose to the CoHS dean that the SON dean submit all proposed decisions to the CoHS associate dean (and when appropriate, to the CoHS dean) allowing 72 hours for comment. If no comment is received within 72 hours, the SON dean will assume the SON can move forward with its decision The SON dean will defer to the CoHS dean in all university meetings
SON chair	The SON chair will coordinate with the CoHS associate dean and other CoHS staff, as appropriate to issues that arise. The chair will apprise the SON dean of the results of these interactions
SON associate chair	The SON associate chair will ensure that all SON publications and official letters include letterhead with the CoHS taking precedence above the SON letterhead and logo – to demonstrate that the SON is a school within the CoHS
Program directors	The program directors will ensure that students and faculty within their programs make every effort to collaborate with the CoHS faculty and students – to demonstrate that the SON is a "team player"

Box 9.9 Key Points to Consider
- The problem/issue is a highly sensitive one.
- While a simpler approach to resolution might initially seem preferable, it will not lead to the best solution.
- Red Team approaches lead to the best solution because all pertinent perspectives are involved.

The SON dean also recognizes that the politics of an academic institution is not solely defined by written duties and responsibilities. That, as a newcomer trying to be innovative and move the SON forward, her assertiveness on behalf of the SON has been regarded as a challenge to the CoHS. Her first priority needs to be building trust with the CoHS by accepting that she must move slowly to build relationships. After faith and trust are established, she can move fast.

Critical Thinking Questions

1. Why is it important in this case to include the entire SON as one stakeholder?
2. What is the advantage of involving all SON faculty and staff in these exercises?
3. Why did not the SON dean include the CoHS dean in these Red Team exercises?

Conflict Between the Front- and Back-Office Staff at Purple Clinic

10

Issue/Problem Purple Clinic is a community health clinic located in the heart of an urban underserved neighborhood. It provides primary care and a few specialty services to people without insurance. The staff is small but there are conflicts between the front-office and the clinical staff with regard to several of the processes used to receive and discharge patients.

Background Purple Clinic has been serving this neighborhood and the county for 15 years. There is one full-time primary care provider, one full-time registered nurse, and one full-time medical assistant who provide clinical services. Various specialists offer weekly volunteer hours. A few volunteer translators assist the clinicians because the patients are primarily immigrants from a variety of countries. The front-office staff includes an executive director, an assistant director, a receptionist who also assists with medical referrals, and an additional staff member who rotates as needed to support the office staff. These personnel work full time and have non-medical backgrounds. There is a paid part-time medical director who is a retired physician. He assists with administration and sees a few patients every week.

Solving the Problem The executive director and the medical director have determined that the conflict between clinical back-office staff and non-clinical front-office staff has reached a point that is impacting workflow and quality of worklife for everyone in the clinic. The executive director was introduced to Red Teaming at a recent management conference and decides to use Red Teaming methods to solve the problems. For the purposes of demonstrating how one might employ a variety of Red Team methods, we will separate the problems and approach them separately. The first issue pertains to scheduling appointments. Box 10.1 lists the Red Team tools used to work through the first issue.

© The Author(s), under exclusive license to Springer Nature Switzerland AG 2021   93
L. Neal-Boylan, S. Rotkoff, *Innovative Decision Making in Healthcare*,
https://doi.org/10.1007/978-3-030-72648-5_10

> **Box 10.1 Red Team Tools Used to Work Through the First Issue**
> - 5 whys.
> - My 15%.
> - 5 will get you 25.
> - Second chance meeting.

Issue #1: **Scheduling Appointments**

The executive director recognizes that the first step is to *better understand the problem*. She and the medical director gather the front-office staff after work one day to try the *5 whys* approach.

The conversation evolves like this:

- *Why 1*: Why is there a conflict between you and the back-office staff?
- Answer: There is a conflict because the back-office staff is always complaining.
- *Why 2*: Why do you think the back-office staff is always complaining?
- Answer: They say they have too many patients to manage each day.
- *Why 3*: Why do they think they have too many patients to manage?
- Answer: They say we do not make appointments based on why the patient is coming in to see the Nurse Practitioner (NP).
- *Why 4*: Why do not you schedule appointments based on the reason the patient is coming in?
- Answer: Because we do not know how long it is going to take the NP to see each type of problem.
- *Why 5*: Why do not you know how long it is going to take the NP to see each type of problem?
- Answer: Because no one has ever explained that to us.

The executive director and the medical director conduct the *5 whys* with the back-office staff on another day after work. Their conversation follows:

- *Why 1*: Why is there a conflict between you and the front-office staff?
- Answer: There is a conflict because the front-office staff does not schedule appointments according to how much time we need to see them.
- *Why 2*: Why is it the responsibility of the front-office staff to judge how long it will take you to see patients?
- Answer: Because they schedule the patients and make the appointments. They tell the patients what time to arrive.
- *Why 3*: Why don't they take the length of time needed into consideration when scheduling the appointments?
- Answer: Because they do not have a clear understanding of the time required for the various different appointments.

- *Why 4*: Why don't they have the understanding required?
- Answer: Because we do not have a process or guideline to help them include the appointment time associated with the most prevalent types of appointments.

Conducting the 5 *whys* with each group eventually resulted in arriving at similar answers. The front-office staff does not know how much time is needed for each type of patient complaint and the back-office staff has not provided this information.

To *change the frame* (Chap. 3) the directors then ask the entire staff to consider *My 15%* (Chap. 3). Specifically, they ask each person to consider what they can do to fix the problem. Index cards are distributed so each staff member can jot down their thoughts. Everyone is given 10 minutes for this exercise. The directors then bring the large group together, and each person is given the opportunity to share what they think they can do to fix the problem without additional resources or changes in policy.

After each individual has written down their 15% the compiled list looks like this:

Front-Office List

I can:

1. Put together a list based on my experience with patients of how long I think appointments generally take and then ask the medical staff to review and correct the list.
2. Ask more detailed questions when scheduling an appointment to better appreciate whether the patient has complications beyond the reasons for their visit that might extend the appointment.
3. Ask the medical staff when I am uncertain of the expected length of an appointment before scheduling it.
4. Start my own log, noting the expected time for an appointment versus the actual time, so that over the course of several weeks, my ability to predict appointment length will improve.

Back-Office List

I can:

1. Put together a list (with my peers) of how long on average an appointment for the most common visits usually take.
2. Put together a list of questions the appointment staff can ask to identify common and appointment extending complications associated with each ailment and the amount of time for which they should extend the appointment.
3. Build flex time into the schedule to allows us to either extend an appointment without disrupting the day, or if available, use that flex time in a designated and useful way to complete other work.
4. Make myself more available and less intimidating to the front-office staff.

As a result of these exercises, the clinical staff in the back office take responsibility for developing a list of the most common reasons people come to the clinic for care and how long the average patient with each problem should need for a visit. The front-office staff commits to asking the clinical staff if they are unsure of how long a particular patient visit will take before they book the appointment.

Using the *5 will get you 25* approach, the executive director invites each of the volunteer specialists (5) to join the larger group. The large group now consists of 12 people. She asks each person to use an index card to note what they think will be the biggest challenge to implementing this new system. Each person receives a different colored card with a matching pen. Recall from Chap. 3, the directions required to use this approach correctly (Box 10.2).

The executive director then asks each person to circulate around the room handing their index card (text side up) to someone else. In turn, each person keeps handing the index card they receive to another person in the room until the director says "STOP." Once everyone has received a card that is not their own (it is a different color), the director tells each person to read the card and determine the quality of the idea. A great idea is given a 5, a good idea a 4, terrible ideas a 1, poor or mediocre ideas a 2 or 3, respectively. Each person writes the number they think fits the idea on the back of the card.

Then, everyone circulates around the room again, rotating cards with the text side up (so no one can see the number ranking on the back side of the card). When the director says "STOP," each person reads the idea on the card but does not rank the idea until they are certain this is not their own card or one they have already ranked. Once that is certain, the director permits everyone to add the grade they think appropriate to the back of the card.

With 12 people in the group, the executive director decides to conduct the rotation one more time (see Chap. 3). She then has everyone return to their seats to determine if any of the challenges identified on the card they have, ranked a 4 or above. (These are the challenges identified anonymously through this approach that are of concern to the most people.)

The group identifies the most significant challenges to implementing the new appointment system as:

• Creating a list that will apply to most patients since all patients have individual needs even though their diagnoses may be similar.

- Maintaining the list.
- Remembering to refer to the list when scheduling appointments.

Having identified these challenges, the director assigns each group of office staff the following responsibilities:

- The back-office staff will create a list of the most common appointment needs and the time associated for each appointment.
- They will also create a list of questions for the front office to ask to determine whether there should be adjustments to the base appointment times. For example:
  - Do you have diabetes? If yes, add 3 minutes to the appointment.
  - Do you smoke? If yes, add 2 minutes.
  - Do you have high blood pressure? If not, deduct 2 minutes.
- The front-office teams will develop procedures to maintain and update their list as questions arise.
- Develop methods to ensure the list is used when making appointments.

A few weeks later, the executive director brings the group of 12 back together and utilizes the *second chance meeting* approach to evaluate the new system. Each person is given an index card and asked to anonymously write whether the new system improved or resolved the problem and why or why not. The executive director collects the cards and reads them aloud. She uses a white board to record the responses and encourages an open discussion. The challenges that were initially identified have been managed with varying degrees of success.

Based on the feedback from the *second chance meeting*, the facilitator helps the group determine the best practices that have worked. Then the group addresses system modifications that have been most difficult to implement. The result is refinement and streamlining and a system that is better than that the group originally implemented (having harvested the best ideas), but still not perfect. The group agrees to come together again in 2 weeks and continue the refinement process. This continues until the group is mostly satisfied with the procedure that is then codified and part of the on-boarding process for new employees (see Box 10.3 for more key points to consider).

Box 10.3 More Key Points to Consider
- The front-office and back-office staff must work well together to ensure a smooth process for staff and patients.
- It is important to better understand the problem before trying to change the frame.
- The second chance meeting approach allows everyone to evaluate the process. This allows everyone to commit to implementing a solution without feeling they are stuck with it if it does not work.

Issue #2: Screening Patients for COVID 19

The clinical staff have complained that the front office is not adequately screening patients to see if they might have the COVID 19 virus before scheduling an appointment. The clinical staff report to the medical director that the front-office staff are supposed to ask every patient specific questions over the phone to assess whether the patient might have been exposed to the virus or might have the virus. However, patients have been checked in and put into exam rooms only to find that they have been exposed to the virus or have symptoms.

Solving the Problem: The executive director and the medical director confer and determine that this is a complex problem (See *Cynefin Framework,* Chap. 4). It is a complex problem because the COVID 19 virus can be asymptomatic and because patients might not know if they have been exposed to the virus. (See Box 10.4 for Red Team tools used to resolve issue number two). The current screening system is designed as if COVID 19 is a simple problem. As a consequence, the leadership decides they need to revisit their procedures in a way that recognizes the complexity of the problem. This requires soliciting divergent ideas to build a better process.

Once again, the directors bring the clinical staff (including the medical specialists) and front-office staff together and use *think-write-share*(T-W-S) (Chap. 3) to find out more about their perspectives. Members of the group pair off (randomly) and share their concerns with their partner. Box 10.5 lists the concerns shared by the groups of two to the larger group.

Box 10.4 Red Team Tools to Work Through Issue #2
- Think-write-hare.
- 1-2-4-all.
- Yes, and….

Box 10.5 Concerns About Issue #2
- Patients are asked screening questions when they call for an appointment, but we frequently leave voice messages to remind people of their appointments and a week or more may pass between the screening questions and the actual appointment.
- Patients are checked in and installed in the exam room before we triage them and find out they have been exposed to COVID or do not feel well.
- By the time the patient is in the exam room, they have been exposed to the people at the front desk, those in the waiting room, and the back-office staff, as well as interpreters in some cases.
- We have to tell these patients we cannot see them and they have to walk through the clinic to leave.

- We do not test them in the clinic so they may expose themselves to others after they leave.
- We should not turn patients away unless it is very likely they have the virus. We need to bring in as many patients as possible or will lose our funding.

Box 10.6 Proposed Solutions
1. The front office should remind patients of the restrictions for entering the clinic when they remind patients of their appointments.
2. In addition to taking their temperature, patients should be asked the screening questions again before they are allowed into the clinic.
3. The front-office staff should direct patients to a COVID testing site.
4. Patients who think they might have symptoms of COVID should be offered a telehealth visit rather than an in-person visit. We can charge for this and also protect our staff and patients.
5. All staff, including front-office staff, should wear PPE during work hours.

The directors then employ the *1-2-4-all* approach. The executive director places two groups of two together into one group of four. With a total of 12 people, this results in 3 groups of four. The groups are asked to discuss these concerns and propose a solution. Once each group has reached a proposed solution, the spokesperson for each group rotates to another group and shares the proposed solution. Each of the groups uses the *Yes, and...* approach to augment or enhance the proposed solution.

At the conclusion of this exercise, the large group re-forms and the medical director facilitates as the spokespeople share the refined solutions from their own groups. Box 10.6 lists the proposed solutions.

The front- and back-office staff agree to implement these solutions. Everyone expresses relief at the measures that are likely to offer them better protection against the COVID virus. The front-office staff accepts that the solutions would require more time from them, but they verbalize that the time would be worth a higher level of reassurance. All agree to use the *second chance meeting* system in 2 weeks to revisit the problem and proposed solutions.

The two issues described in the case of the Purple Clinic are examples of issues that are typical of an outpatient community clinic. Using Red Team approaches, staff, volunteers, and directors reached viable solutions that everyone agreed to attempt. Everyone had a say in analyzing the problems and proposing solutions.

Critical Thinking Questions

1. Did the *5 whys* clarify the issue better than a standard approach?
2. Why was the *1-2-4-all* approach an important sequela to the T-W-S method?
3. How does *yes, and...* enhance the proposed solutions?

Hierarchy at Blue University School of Nursing

11

Problem/Issue Blue University is a large public university that is experiencing significant financial difficulties.

Background The School of Nursing (SON) is the largest school in the university and is the second highest revenue generator. The university counts on the SON to contribute significant revenue to help keep the other schools and non-revenue-producing departments afloat. The dean and the school of nursing finance officer have reviewed the budget and think money can be saved in a variety of ways. These include reduction of travel expenses, increasing faculty workload, and reducing the use of simulation to teach students.

Solving the Problem The dean asks for volunteers to comprise an ad hoc committee to study the issue. The finance officer will sit on the committee as an advisor and a staff member will schedule the meetings and take minutes. The volunteer members include three senior faculty who are tenured full professors and happen to be the sole members of the SON Promotion and Tenure committee. Other committee members include two junior faculty who are new to academe. The dean gives the committee its charge: To find a way to save costs without layoffs. She then leaves the committee to conduct its business and awaits the committee's report and recommendations due in 3 months.

Part One

The committee holds its first meeting and one of the tenured professors (Neesha) quickly assumes the role of committee chair. She declares that the meetings will occur every other week and last an hour. Neesha's first request is that the finance officer (Libby) give the committee a detailed accounting of how much money the SON spends per year on travel, adjunct (part-time) faculty, and simulation. Once the committee has these data, they begin to discuss the choices given them by the dean. Each faculty member contributes to the discussion about each option, but the external conversations they present to the committee members are different from their internal conversations – what they need and want for themselves. The faculty begin by discussing option one: Travel reimbursement. (See Box 11.1 for key points to consider).

Option One

External Dialogue

Neesha (tenured professor) says she spends a lot of time traveling to conferences to present her research. She worries that the school's reputation will suffer if she and other faculty cannot attend conferences.

Eleanor, (assistant professor) new to the faculty, chimes in that she thinks many faculty attend conferences to keep current with the profession and nursing education. To not attend would impact the cutting-edge education they pride themselves on giving to the students.

Eli, (tenured full professor), says that attending conferences is a time-honored tradition among academics and is necessary to the faculty role.

Christopher, (assistant professor), points out that there is clinical travel as well as conference travel. Faculty must make visits to clinical sites where students are placed. Faculty are reimbursed per mile traveled and often submit meal receipts for reimbursement.

Libby refers to her spreadsheet and notes that several hundred thousand dollars per year is spent on reimbursement of faculty clinical site visits and conference attendance.

Easton, (tenured full professor), says that he no longer makes clinical site visits and that he rarely attends conferences anymore.

Internal Dialogue

Neesha: I enjoy going to conferences. I get the opportunity to network but also to reconnect with old friends. Sometimes, the conferences are located where there are clothing stores we do not have at home. Conferences take me away from the day-to-day stresses of my job.

Eleanor: I am trying to get recognized in nursing education, and I want to mix with the movers and shakers in nursing education. They always attend these conferences. I want them to get to know me. I do not plan to be at Blue University forever. I am already planning my path to promotion and my next move.

Eli: I am getting ready to retire so I really do not care too much about tradition. But as senior faculty, I think we have earned the right to decide whether or not I want to travel.

Christopher: These site visits are a good deal. I get to keep the reimbursement for mileage, but the cost of the gas I use in my car is cheaper than what I use on any one of these trips. I get money for a meal, but I rarely use it or spend as much as I am allotted. I am making money on these visits, and I make a lot of visits every semester.

> **Box 11.1 Key Points to Consider**
> - Senior, tenured faculty have little to lose and a lot to gain.
> - Junior non-tenured faculty have a lot to lose and a lot to gain.
> - Everyone has a vested interest in a particular solution.

Easton: Between my 2 days working clinically and my family life, I have no interest in travel.

Option Two

During the next meeting, the members discuss option two: An increase in faculty workload. Previously, the dean pointed out that most full-time faculty are teaching six credits per semester but are not publishing or presenting any research or scholarship. Typically, faculty would be expected to use the remaining three to six credits per semester to conduct research and publish or engage in some other form of scholarship. Not only are faculty not engaging in scholarship or disseminating their findings, but adjunct faculty must be hired to teach the courses faculty are unavailable to teach because of their reduced credit load. Libby calculates that several hundred thousand dollars are spent on hiring adjuncts per year.

External Dialogue

Easton comments that faculty at Blue University SON have had this workload for a long time, and it would be very disruptive to change it. He emphasizes that the faculty are excellent teachers and board exam scores are high so there is no need for change.

Neesha concurs stating that adjunct faculty bring real-world and current expertise to nursing education, and if they are not utilized, students will miss out on this expertise and the adjuncts might seek work in other universities and not be available in the future. She says, "The system we have exists for a reason."

Internal Dialogue

Easton: I enjoy my workload of six credits each semester. I have teenagers at home. I like getting home early most days and being on campus only 2 days a week, most weeks. This allows me to work in my own clinical practice as a Nurse Practitioner 2 days a week, and I keep the money I earn on top of my academic salary. I am not interested in doing any research. I was tenured before any of that was required. I only have a few more years until I can retire. I do not want to start working harder now.

Neesha: There is no way I intend to teach additional classes. I have worked hard to gain seniority and not have to teach clinicals. I serve on several committees. That is enough.

Options one and two are discussed extensively at subsequent meetings and then Neesha decides to spend time discussing the last option presented by the dean – to reduce the use of simulation to instruct students.

External Dialogue

Eleanor reminds everyone that clinical placements for students are hard to find, and there is a lot of competition among the nursing schools in the area for clinical experiences for students. Simulated clinical practice provides students with much needed experience in a safe environment where they can make mistakes and not hurt anyone.

Christopher agrees with this and comments that students and faculty enjoy the simulated experiences.

Eli points out that simulation is now a major part of nursing education today, and other schools of nursing will think less of the SON at Blue University if simulation is reduced.

Internal Dialogue

Eleanor: Most of my workload involves teaching simulation. What will happen if we reduce how much we use it? They will assign me to classes I do not want to teach. I am new, maybe they will make me go down to part-time.

Christopher: I was hoping to become an expert in simulation. I am trying to work my way into teaching simulation and convincing my supervisor to send me to a training conference in simulation. That is not likely if we do not need as many instructors who know how to teach simulation.

Eli: I am in charge of the simulation lab and everyone defers to me about anything that has to do with simulation. I have not worked in clinical practice for a long time, so what would I teach if they reduced simulation? Would I still be in charge?

Outcome

After a series of meetings, the committee is unable to reach a decision and the deadline to give the dean a report is nearing. The senior faculty, Neesha, Eli, and Easton convene prior to the next meeting and decide they will vote to place restrictions on conference travel. They agree that faculty requests to attend conferences should be scored based on faculty rank, years at the university, and whether or not they are presenting a paper or poster at the conference. The senior faculty are the majority on the committee, and their vote carries the day. Senior faculty are assured of being able to continue to attend conferences. The junior faculty on the committee are disappointed but hide their feelings about the unfairness of the decision.

Box 11.2 Red Team Tools Used in This Case
- Think-write-share.
- Round Robin.
- Dot voting.
- TRIZ.

Part Two

The remainder of this case presents the issue and resolution using a Red Team approach. A large part of the challenge of this committee will be to escape preconceived perspectives of the different committee members and ensure the best idea among the many options wins. Use of Red Team tools will enable this committee to overcome bias and separate the best ideas from those held by the most senior members of the committee.

Using the Red Team approach, an additional member will be added to the committee. This is a person who has been trained in Red Team techniques and who will facilitate committee discussions; however, this new member, Paul, will not be substantively involved in the nature of what is discussed. In other words, he will be an impartial facilitator. Box 11.2 lists the Red Team tools used in this case. Paul has a wide variety of Red Team tools at his disposal. Like a golfer, he ponders what the right club is for this specific situation. He begins with the tool *think-write-share* (Chap. 3).

Paul asks everyone to think very carefully and reflectively about the problem. He instructs them to block out distractions and think hard for a full 5 minutes, considering the problem of the need to cut the SON budget. He requests they list the pros and cons of each of the three options (cutting travel expenses, increasing faculty workload, using less simulation). He then asks everyone to write down their thoughts without self-censoring.

After everyone looks up indicating they have finished writing, Paul then employs a second Red Teaming tool: *Round Robin* (Chap. 3). He asks each person to share one idea from their own list. Paul records the ideas on a white board making two columns (pros and cons). No one speaks twice until everyone has had a chance to speak once. As each person hears an idea they had on their list, they cross it off their list. Round Robin continues until everyone has completed their list.

A couple of new ideas beyond cutting travel expenses, increasing faculty workload, and using less simulation have appeared on the list. However, Paul explains these cannot be included because the dean stipulated three possible alternatives. He suggests these additional alternatives be added to the final proposal to the dean as options to consider, but the remainder of the meetings will only focus on the initial three options.

Paul refers to the list of ideas on the white board to employ the *dot voting* strategy. He asks each person to put a colored dot on the item on the list (travel expenses, increasing faculty workload, and reducing the use of simulation to teach students) they think should be the strategy for reducing costs. Paul then takes the item with the most votes and prepares for the next step, *TRIZ*. (Since there are only five people in the group, more than one option may receive a majority of dot votes. Consequently, Paul will conduct another round of dot voting with only these two options, forcing a majority to vote for one option).

To use TRIZ, Paul divides the group of five into two groups, mixing them so they include both senior and junior faculty. He asks each group to design ways in which the chosen item (travel expenses, increasing faculty workload, or reducing the use of simulation to teach students) can fail. Robust discussion follows. He then brings the larger group together and records these reasons on the white board. The larger group discusses whether the likelihood of failing can be mitigated or whether each option must be discarded and replaced with a different option. The final proposal is prepared for submission to the dean. The large group works together to list the rationale for the proposal.

Outcome

The proposal submitted to the dean includes a combination of approaches. The outcome of using the Red Team strategies is that a combination will ensure that neither junior nor senior faculty get priority. The proposal includes less reliance on adjunct faculty, more circumspection about travel (who is presenting a paper, who has a role within the SON that requires they keep current in a certain topical area, etc.), and an increase in faculty workload based on whether faculty are research active (publish one article per year), productive (publish at least three articles per year), or intensive (have steady grant funding for their research).

The committee also includes approaches beyond the three suggested by the dean, such as increasing fundraising within the SON and critically reviewing curricula to determine if the SON should begin a new program that will bring in additional funds while cutting programs that bring in little revenue.

Use of the Red Team tools required the committee members to consider ways to save money, despite their vested interests and precludes any attempt to try and shape the outcome in their own favor. Using these Red Team approaches prevented an "all or nothing" outcome. Smart efficiencies and savings are more likely to be uncovered and discussed. Also, requiring people to first work independently and then in structured collaboration, prevented the senior faculty from taking control of the committee and achieving what is in their own best interest to the possible detriment of the junior faculty.

Critical Thinking Questions

1. What is (are) the real issues in this case?
2. How does consideration of both internal and external dialogues help in the analysis of this case?
3. How did the outcome differ using the Red Team approaches versus without the Red Team approaches?
4. Did Red Team approaches lead to the best idea winning?

What to Build at Turquoise University School of Nursing

12

Issue/Problem Turquoise University School of Nursing (SON) has been tasked with raising capital funds to build a new wing that will most likely house all the simulation and health assessment labs.

Background While simulation has become a core component of nursing curricula, the SON dean believes it is crucial to plan for 5 years into the future and beyond. After several discussions with the provost and chief financial officer, the SON dean realizes he has a few choices as he plans for the new building:

1. Build a mini hospital including simulation rooms, debriefing rooms, state-of-the-art health assessment labs, and a mock operating room (OR) for the Certified Registered Nurse Anesthesia (CRNA) program.
2. Build a mini hospital that will include simulation rooms, and debriefing rooms but continue to have CRNA students acquire all their OR practice in area hospitals.
3. Leave the simulation and debriefing rooms as they are now and use the new building for new classrooms and faculty offices.

Solving the Problem The SON dean requests a Red Team consultant, Andrew, to help with this process. The dean meets privately with Andrew to discuss his vision. Together, they decide that how they arrived at the decision is as important as the actual decision and that the dean needs faculty support and advocacy for whichever decision emerges from the Red Team process. With this in mind, they decide on the following macro approach:

1. Create a shared vision of Turquoise University SON 5 years from now. This vision will form the foundation of any subsequent examination of whether or not to build. The current SON strategic plan is due to expire in 2 years and does not include a plan for a new building.

© The Author(s), under exclusive license to Springer Nature Switzerland AG 2021
L. Neal-Boylan, S. Rotkoff, *Innovative Decision Making in Healthcare*,
https://doi.org/10.1007/978-3-030-72648-5_12

Box 12.1 Red Team Tools Used in This Case
- Forced distribution.
- Second chance meeting.
- What-if analysis.
- Think-write-share.
- Ad Agency.
- Best of breed.
- Pre-mortem analysis.

2. Examine alternative futures to ensure the decision made today is developed in recognition of factors the SON cannot control.
3. Based on a common vision and an understanding of the vagaries of the future, build a list of advantages and disadvantages of each option and then make a recommendation to the provost and chief financial officer. Box 12.1 lists the Red Team tools used to resolve this case.

Session One

Session one focuses on creating a shared vision of Turquoise University SON 5 years hence.

Each member of the faculty is asked to write a vision statement, individually and anonymously describing the SON 5 years hence. Their descriptions need to include how the SON and the nursing profession might look different than today, be clear and concise (no longer than three sentences), and be restricted to a single side of a 4 × 6 index card.

Faculty are told to aim for tangible descriptions, not lovely words describing unmeasurable qualities. They are instructed to write this vision on an index card in block lettering to separate the source of the vision statement from the perceived quality of that statement. They are instructed not to discuss their vision statement with anyone else.

Once the vision statements are completed, they are collected and mixed up to maintain anonymity. Then all of the statements are placed on the wall of the room. The group is then told to review the visions and apply a *forced distribution* grading criteria (Chap. 3) to them. In this case, since there are 21 participants and 21 vision statements; participants are told they can hand out seven grades of 9 or 10, seven grades of 7 or 8, and a minimum of seven grades of 6 and below. Each person is given a piece of paper on which to anonymously record a grade for each index card describing a vision.

Faculty turn the grades in to Andrew who tabulates them. He reads aloud the top three visions and the common themes captured by the group. Following that, Andrew reads other visions looking specifically for ideas not already included in the top three.

> **Box 12.2 Homework to Prepare for Session Two**
> - Identify the three things you fear the most that are outside your control that would affect the future of the school.
> - Identify the three assumptions about school performance that are most critical to future success.
>
> Give your answers back to the facilitator without sharing with the rest of the group.

The group works together to build the best vision statement from the highest ranking three statements. By the end of the conversation, the faculty have a vision statement on which they can all agree. Finally, Andrew leads them through a *second chance meeting* exercise in which everyone is asked to anonymously affirm that they agree with and can support the vision statement. Once this is accomplished, Andrew assigns homework for session two (Box 12.2). Prior to assigning the homework, he provides an introduction to the preparatory work. Andrew explains there are two general categories of things that can dramatically affect future planning. They are as follows:

1. Things we cannot control, such as the national economy, demographic trends, and government policy.
2. Things we can control but make assumptions about as we plan, such as the level of fundraising, our competition, and what we offer as a school.

Andrew sends the answers back to the faculty for another anonymous vote prior to session two. The faculty respond that their greatest fears/things that cannot be controlled are the following:

- National economy
- National enrollment trends

The faculty respond that the three assumptions most critical to future success are the following:

- Fundraising
- SON initiatives
- Size, scope, timing of building project

Session Two

Session two is divided into parts.

Part One

Andrew determines that the first approach, given the fears expressed by the faculty is a *What-if* analysis. He uses a white board to draw the graphic below (Fig. 12.1):

Andrew explains that the upper right quadrant represents the best-case scenario. The lower left quadrant represents the worst-case scenario. The areas in between represent suboptimal cases that are based on different sets of circumstances. It is important when using this tool that the X-axis and Y-axis represent independent variables. While a weak economy might reduce enrollment, it is not the main reason the faculty fear declining enrollment. They are concerned that enrollment could decline for several reasons unrelated to the economy:

- Post COVID-19 virus education at brick and mortar institutions might be less popular.
- The COVID 19 virus might discourage people from entering the nursing profession for fear of exposure to dangerous diseases.
- There have been and are likely to be demographic reductions in college-age students.
- There are changes in the size of the local population.

Andrew breaks the faculty into four groups: Three groups of five people and one group of six people. He asks each group to fill out the following form for their assigned quadrant (Table 12.1):

Initially, Andrew assigns each group to a quadrant, based on the graph in Fig. 12.1. They start with the *think-write-share* (T-W-S) exercise, confer within their group, and fill in the chart. Next, the groups are mixed to facilitate further creative thought in the groups. Finally, Andrew assembles everyone into one large group to summarize the progress. Box 12.3 offers an example of how this might occur for one of the quadrants: Best case.

Fig. 12.1 What-if analysis

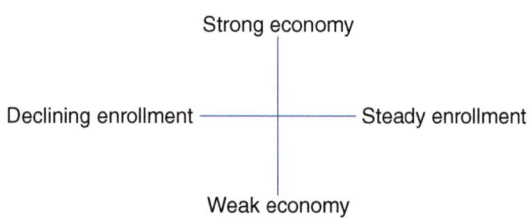

Table 12.1 Form to complete for each quadrant

	Advantages	Disadvantages
Mini hospital with OR		
Mini hospital without OR		
Classrooms and offices		

Box 12.3 Quadrant Analysis for the Best-Case Scenario – Strong Economy and Steady Enrollment

Choice #1: Build a mini hospital including the simulation rooms, debriefing rooms, and a mock operating room for the Certified Registered Nurse Anesthesia (CRNA) program:

Advantages: We will attract students who want to benefit from the latest in cutting-edge technology in nursing education; our CRNA students will be better prepared when they begin their clinical rotations; local hospitals can use our OR to orient and train OR staff; prospective nursing students and their families are likely to be impressed by the facilities and that may make them more likely to attend our SON; other health disciplines in the university might find the OR useful for practice.

Disadvantages: Fundraising will be challenging; it will take years to build the mini hospital to include all of these rooms; once the OR is built, we will need special anesthesia/OR equipment that can be expensive; the medical school in the university may decide to compete with us by launching an anesthesia assistant program.

Choice #2: Build a mini hospital that will include simulation rooms, and debriefing rooms but continue to have CRNA students acquire all their OR practice in area hospitals:

Advantages: Save some money and fundraising if exclude OR; still be attractive to potential students; we can open the mini hospital and additional simulation rooms to our community partners to use to orient their staff – this could bring in additional funding; we are more likely to be able to achieve national certification in simulation; we may attract more prestigious faculty; parents of prospective students will be impressed by our mini hospital.

Disadvantages: Our CRNA program will be competing with programs that have mock operating rooms; the clinical placements we have for our CRNA students may not remain robust and we may have fewer sites in which our students can practice.

Choice #3: Leave the simulation and debriefing rooms as there are now and use the new building for new state-of-the-art classrooms and faculty offices:

Advantages: Add sorely needed classroom and office space potentially allowing us to hire new faculty; cheaper than the other two options; we can include the latest in educational technology in the classrooms which is likely to attract prospective students; increase the potential for interprofessional learning if we build smart classrooms.

Disadvantages: We will be behind our competitors in simulation, health assessment lab technology, and in the CRNA program; might limit our ability to hire new faculty and increase the number of tenured and tenure track researchers.

Andrew asks each of the groups to share their quadrant analysis with the entire faculty. Then, each individual is asked to anonymously vote for their choice for each quadrant. Faculty are then asked to imagine themselves in each of the potential future scenarios described by their colleagues in the quadrant analysis. They then vote for one of the three choices regarding the new building (Box 12.3). Box 12.4 shows the tabulation of the votes.

Before moving on to part two, it is important to review the key considerations in this case (Box 12.5).

Box 12.4 Tabulation of the Votes

Upper right quadrant (best case – strong economy, steady enrollment): Choice #1–10 votes; Choice #2–8 votes; Choice #3–3 votes.

Upper left quadrant (medium case – weak economy declining enrollment): Choice #1–5 votes; Choice #2–12 votes; Choice #3–4 votes.

Bottom right quadrant (medium case – steady enrollment, Strong economy): Choice #1–2 votes; Choice #2–17 votes; Choice #3–2 votes.

Bottom left quadrant (medium case – steady enrollment, weak economy): Choice #1–8 votes: Choice #2–12 votes; Choice #3–1 vote.

Box 12.5 Key Considerations in This Case
- SONs should always be thinking of the impact of the future of the nursing profession and healthcare when planning.
- Building projects are multi-year, multi-phase efforts and require careful planning and consideration.
- Red Teaming lends itself to futuristic thinking and planning because it engages multiple perspectives, not just higher administration.
- Red Teaming invites and encourages innovative thinking that can significantly and positively affect plans for the future.

Part Two

Having addressed the most prevalent fears about the future, the group focuses on the most critical assumptions. There are 21 people in the group and three critical assumptions that were expressed through anonymous feedback so Andrew chooses to use the *Ad Agency* approach. (See Box 12.6 for a note regarding choice of Red Team tools).

Refer to the *Ad Agency* method described in Chapter Four. Three groups are created and each member of the group is given a different charge:

Box 12.6 Choosing Red Team Tools
When selecting a tool to use, facilitators must consider what emerges from the use of the initial tools (in this case, *think-write-share*) to select which tools to use next. For example, if in this case, two critical assumptions had emerged and there were eight people in the large group, one might use *1-2-4 all* as a way of discussing each assumption.

A – Develop ideas around how to optimize fundraising/financing in ways not currently being pursued
B – Consider new initiatives and ways to mitigate risk, if we pursue them
C – Build parameters or ways to mitigate risk around size, scope, and timing
The *Ad Agency* approach is used as described in Chap. 4.
Step 1: **A, B, C** – think and write ideas specific to their charge.
Step 2: **A** shares ideas with **B** and **C.**

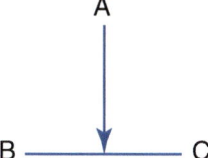

Step 3: **A** walks away and allows B and C to discuss among themselves.

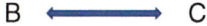

Step 4: **B** and **C** provide feedback to **A.**

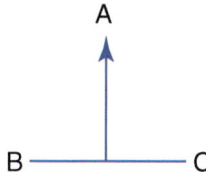

Step 5: Repeat until B and C have gone through the Steps two, three and four.

Step 6: Each group employs the *best of breed* (Chap. 3) approach to come up with the three to five best ideas in each group. Each of the three *best of breed* groups then reports to the entire group. Some of the ideas generated through this process are shown in Box 12.7.

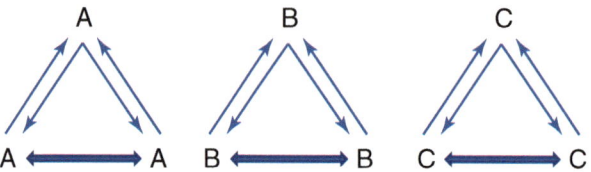

As session two concludes, the SON dean takes responsibility for gathering the feedback and sharing it with the provost and chief financial officer. As a result of using Red Team methods, the SON dean recommends to the provost and chief financial officer that they pursue choice #2 (build a mini hospital that will include simulation rooms, and debriefing rooms but continue to have CRNA students acquire all their OR practice in area hospitals).

Box 12.7 Ideas Generated by Best of Breed Approach

Fund raising

- Approach our clinical partners to contribute.
- Solicit reliable donors to create endowments.
- Hold a special fundraiser or multiple events hosted by our alumni.
- Have low expectations that traditional fundraising will support the scope of building.
- Solicit in-kind contributions by construction companies.

New initiative management

- Create an ad hoc committee to review new ideas and make recommendations to SON.
- Pilot all new ideas versus putting too many resources behind any one initiative.
  Concept of the building

- Involve students in planning.
- Involve community partners and colleagues from across the university in planning.
- Visit other SONs across the country that have successfully raised money and built new buildings to gather input and ideas.
- Build in iterations.
- Begin effective Spring 2022; allow 18 months to get it right.

He shares the work done by the team and the role of Red Team tools and methods in reaching the recommendation (as explained in sessions one and two). Session three is designed for the Office of Advancement and Development (OAD) to approve the measure and develop a funding strategy.

Session Three

After reviewing the recommendation and fielding questions from the OAD, the SON dean turns the session over to the Red Team facilitator, Andrew. The first thing Andrew does is arrange an anonymous *second chance meeting* (Chap. 3). He asks all 10 members of the OAD to approve or disapprove funding choice #2 based on the rationale provided by the SON dean and the answers to their specific questions. They agree choice #2 is worth pursuing further.

During the course of the discussion and exploration of options during sessions one and two, it becomes apparent that the SON cannot raise the money required for the new building through traditional fundraising. They realized that any successful fundraising might decrease the size of their new debt, but ultimately they would either need a bond or a major donor to secure the remaining funds. With those the only options, Andrew decides to use a method called *A Team/ B Team.*

Andrew charges **A** team with making the best possible case for obtaining a bond and the best case against acquiring a major donor. He instructs **B** team to do the opposite: Make a case for a major donor and a case against using bonds. Once the teams have completed their work, the entire group gathers together and each team briefs the large group regarding their arguments for or against. Andrew makes it clear that both teams will be heard in their entirety before the floor is opened for discussion. Team **A** makes their arguments, see Box 12.8.

Team B in its initial discussions arrived at similar conclusions as Team A. But because they were tasked to optimize a solution focused on acquiring a major donor, they came up with a different approach (Box 12.9).

Upon conclusion of this exercise, the OAD recommends a three-tiered strategy for raising the money for the new building:

1. Investigating a bond.
2. Acquiring a major donor.
3. Combining multiple donors who have given significant gifts in the past.

This approach is unanimously adopted. Now that the SON has the outline of a plan (in the next 3 years, to build a mini hospital that will include simulation rooms, and debriefing rooms using a fundraising strategy), it is possible to apply *pre-mortem analysis* (Chap. 4) and test the plan. *Pre-mortem analysis* is a 6-step process (Box 12.10).

Box 12.8 Team A
Bonds are better because of the following:

- The university already has a long-standing relationship with a well-established and friendly lender.
- Currently, rates are historically low.
- The bond holder will not interfere with the decisions the university makes with regard to the buildings, as long as the university can service the loan.

Acquiring a major donor is not desirable because of the following:

- The university assumes all of the risk.
- The donor may want to play a major role in deciding how the building will be designed and the space will be used.
- It will be extremely difficult to get a donor willing to donate such a large amount of money.
- Mixing a major donor with other donors who contribute much less might be a complex task.

Box 12.9 Team B
- Acquiring a major donor only makes sense if the donor has similar goals and values and respects the SON mission and vision.
- Partner with an alumnus who has a history of providing major gifts or has expressed interest in donating a big gift.

All 10 of the OAD members take 10 minutes to conduct Steps 1–3 of the *pre-mortem analysis*. They then move on to Step 4 and share a variety of future failures along with the events that they imagined would lead to that failure. Box 12.11 includes examples of ways in which the plan might fail:

After listening to all 10 individually developed *pre-mortem analyses*, the group moves on to Step 5. It is clear that the two concerns that could make the building initiative a failed venture are a drop in enrollment (whatever the cause) and an inability to service the debt (whatever the cause). With that, Andrew breaks the large group into two teams. The first team (A) is charged with identifying ways to

Box 12.10 Use of Pre-mortem Analysis in This Case
- *Step 1*: Have a plan.
- *Step 2*: Imagine that the plan has failed in some spectacular way in the future. This is the *pre-mortem*. You can, but do not have to have, a specific deadline in mind.
- *Step 3*: Individually, walk backward from the imagined future until the inception of the plan; explain the events that happened to lead to the imagined future.
- *Step 4*: Share your scenario with others on your team.
- *Step 5*: Look for common events or risks across the different pre-mortems. These events can lead up to the same or very different failures.
- *Step 6*: Look for ways to PRECLUDE the event from happening, MONITOR warning signs that the event is happening, and REACT if the event happens.

Box 12.11 Ways in Which the Plan Might Fail
- Prospective nursing student enrollment drops.
- A new administration makes attending college free and small private universities suffer and enrollment drops.
- There is a massive economic downturn and families cannot afford college and enrollment drops.
- Several key personnel in the admissions department leave and enrollment drops.
- There is a massive economic down-turn and the bond holder wants to collect all of the principal and interest so the school cannot make payments on the bond.
- There is a massive economic down-turn and prospective donors no longer want to donate to the school.
- The SON changes curricula or their mission and vision and donors no longer want to donate to the school.

preclude, monitor, and *react* to an inability to service the debt and the second team (B) is charged with identifying ways to *preclude, monitor*, and *react* with a focus on enrollment. Box 12.12 lists the responses of Team A to not being able to service the debt.

Group B responds regarding enrollment (Box 12.13).

Box 12.12 Team A Responses
Preclusion strategies:

- Hire a consultant with experience in designing university simulation and laboratory space.
  - Design for affordability.
  - Build in flexibility of use.
  - Build in energy efficiency.
- Financing issues
  - Design flexibility into the bond.
  - No penalty for early repayment.
  - Minimize the amount we finance.
  - Wait until material costs come down.

Things to monitor:

- Occupancy
  - Profitability.
  - Energy efficiency.
  - Debt to service ratio.

How to react if servicing the debt becomes a problem:

- Develop a back-up plan before starting to build.
- Consider asking community partners to pay to use the simulation and lab space to train their staff.
- Use university reserves to bridge the gap.

At the conclusion of these series of meetings, the OAD is very comfortable with their plan of action. Many of the participants marveled at how they had worked through a difficult decision so quickly and that they had gotten a very diverse group to agree with the way ahead. This case illustrates how Red Team methods can assist planners to work through a complex issue and arrive at the best solution.

Box 12.13 Team B Responses
Preclusion strategies

- Take direct action to reduce the impact of personnel changes in the admissions department.
- Maintain good relationships with donors by communicating regularly and involving them in SON activities.
- Frequently provide fun and accessible opportunities for families to learn about the SON so we will be the school of choice for prospective nursing students.

Things to monitor:

- There are already several metrics to monitor enrollment so there is no need to create new ones.
- Increase our presence at local high schools and invite high school students to observe classes, labs, and simulations to encourage enrollment.

How to react if enrollment drops:

- Launch an aggressive strategy to encourage clinical and community partners to pay to utilize the new labs and simulation rooms.
- Develop/strengthen partnerships with organizations that sell healthcare supplies and equipment to encourage them to use our labs and simulation rooms to advertise their healthcare products.

Critical Thinking Questions

1. How did the use of Red Team tools influence the final solution of this case?
2. In what ways was the resolution of this case preferable to a resolution using standard planning methods?
3. Were there disadvantages to using Red Team tools to resolve this case? If so, what were they and how could they be minimized?

Merging Brown Visiting Nurse Association with Gray Health System

13

Issue/Problem Due to financial constraints, Brown Visiting Nurses Association (VNA), a small long-standing community organization must merge with Gray Health System, a large regional conglomerate. The organizational cultures are vastly different, but the two organizations must come together to work as one.

Background The Brown VNA has been a fixture of the community for more than 25 years. It is led by a master's prepared nurse whose leadership style is one of transparency and approachability. She worked for many years as a home health nurse before taking on the chief nurse position. The VNA is primarily staffed by registered nurses (RNs), home health aides (HHAs), physical therapists (PTs), speech language pathologists (SLPs), and occupational therapists (OTs). Some of the RNs are clinical specialists. There is a nurse manager in each of the two offices. The administration of the VNA includes a chief nurse, a chief financial officer, two nurse site managers, and a board of directors consisting of some nurses, the medical director (a physician), a physician ethicist, several community members from various business backgrounds, and one former patient. The Brown VNA also has a nurse educator, utilization review staff who review documentation and submit visits for reimbursement, secretarial staff, and liaisons who work with hospital discharge planners.

RNs manage most of the patient caseloads. However, most of the patients are receiving intermittent skilled care in their homes by an RN, HHA, and at least one therapist. The interdisciplinary team confers in person monthly or more frequently depending on the patients' needs. They are in frequent email contact to ensure consistency of care.

Each office holds monthly staff meetings in person. These are fairly informal. Each nurse manager is present in the office except when she/he has meetings with the chief nurse or other administrator. The nurse managers are available and accessible to their staff and confer frequently to support their staff. Monthly educational in-services are held at one of the two offices. Most people across both offices know each other and many get together outside of work.

The Gray Health System started as one hospital and has expanded to six in the region. The system has grown quickly and has also purchased several private physician practices. They are competing with a large, very prestigious, and long-standing health system 1 hour away and with several small community hospitals in their own region. Their administrators view the merger with the Brown VNA as a way to add home health services and ensure consistency of care for their hospital patients once they are discharged home. The Brown organization will no longer be a VNA after the merger but will be a department within Gray Health System.

The Gray Health System is run by a chief medical officer (physician), a chief nurse, a chief financial officer, a department of human resources, an office of advancement and development, and a board of directors. There is an education department within each hospital whose job it is to keep clinical staff current. There is a director who coordinates all the education departments across the system. The administration also consists of department heads and a hierarchy of supervisors and directors. Each hospital has its own director who reports to the chief medical officer and the central board of directors. Each department within each hospital has a supervisor. Each physician practice is run by a physician who reports to a supervisor directly under the chief medical officer. The health system is widespread and large so staff typically only know the people with whom they interact most often. These are people in their own departments or people with whom they interact on behalf of their patients.

Solving the Problem   Natalie, the chief nurse at Brown VNA, recognizes that significant adjustment will be required for her staff to adapt to the culture of the Gray Health System. She recognizes that while this change is called a merger, the VNA is actually being swallowed up by the Gray Health System. She understands this must happen and was part of the team that made the decision to move ahead with the merger. However, she is realistic that the VNA will need to adopt the culture of the Gray Health System, not the other way around. She sees her task as trying to make the adaptation to the new culture as painless as possible for her staff. In addition, she has decided to retire 1 year following the merger and is aware that the new chief administrator of the VNA will not be a nurse, nor any type of health professional. That person has already been chosen by the health system and is from a business background. Natalie has been asked to mentor the new chief until she retires. See Box 13.1 for key considerations in this case.

> **Box 13.1 Key Considerations**
> - Brown VNA is a relatively small, long-standing organization. Everyone knows each other and they get things done via good communication and their relationships.
> - The Gray Health System has grown quickly, and it is likely most people do not know each other across the system.

- The cultures are very different.
- Brown VNA wants to keep the feeling of closeness and collegiality.
- Gray Health System, by virtue of its size and rapid growth, cannot sustain a culture of closeness throughout the system, but it can cultivate it and sustain it among people who frequently work together.
- The VNA staff are not happy about the merger; that makes this change potentially more difficult on everyone.

Natalie has asked the merger team if she can bring in a consultant to assist with helping the VNA staff begin to adapt to the changes. This request is approved so she brings in Sara who will conduct Red Teaming exercises in each VNA office. After meeting with Natalie and with the VNA board of directors, Sara develops a plan and considers the Red Team tools she will use in this case (Box 13.2).

Box 13.2 Red Team Tools Used in This Case
- Think-write-share (T-W-S).
- My 15%.
- Pre-mortem analysis.

Natalie invites the two nurse site managers, the VNA staff educator, one RN, one PT, one OT, one SLP, and one HHA to attend. She also includes the former patient who sits on the board of directors. The Gray Health System supports this effort and is invested in a smooth merger of organizational cultures. The chief medical officer suggests the chief nurse, the future director of Brown VNA (after Natalie retires), and the director of human resources (HR) also participate. Sara recommends the group meet once a week to Red Team.

During the first session, she leads the group in a *T-W-S* exercise. She asks everyone to consider metrics within their own areas that would indicate that the two cultures have merged successfully. For example, the two nurse site managers consider their own interactions with the future merged administration and the interaction of their staff and what they might expect if the merging of cultures is successful. The VNA staff educator considers how the merger will impact staff education. Each of the clinicians (RN, PT, OT, SLP, HHA) considers how clinical processes might look and how they might interact in interdisciplinary ways if the merger is successful. The former patient thinks about how the cultural change might impact patients, if at all and what would be signs of success. After everyone has had a chance to think and write on their own, Sara collects their notes and lists metrics on a white board. She does not include duplicates. She does not mention who listed which metric. She encourages everyone to discuss these metrics. Box 13.3 lists some of the metrics that emerge from the *T-W-S* exercise.

Box 13.3 Metrics

Natalie (VNA Chief Nurse): Ability to get approvals from system administrators without bureaucratic complexities. Seamless budget discussions and approvals. There is no lag time. We receive approvals within the same timeframe as we do now. Staff retention.

Nurse Site Managers: (same as above), an office environment of people who are happy to be at work and continue to have good working relationships with one another. No changes in how the nurse managers assign patients or support staff. No problem recruiting or hiring staff.

Clinicians: It is important that the incoming chief understand the needs of clinicians. Our managers will advocate for us, but they must have a direct line to the new chief so we can have our needs met appropriately and on time. There should be opportunities for us to meet and socialize with our new clinical partners in the health system, especially those with whom we will communicate most often on behalf of patient care. Processes should not be significantly or quickly changed. We need time to adjust to the merger of organizations. There should be in-services and time off from patient visits to attend the in-services to learn about organizational changes. Surveys from clinicians assessing organizational climate demonstrate people are adjusting to the changes.

Former VNA Patient: Patients should not see a difference in the quality of care they receive. It is already very good. We should be able to benefit from greater consistency of care. Since we will be cared for by one health system, we should be able to trust our medical information will transition smoothly after a hospital stay or from our primary care provider's office to the VNA. Surveys to patients should indicate satisfaction with services.

VNA Staff Educator: The VNA staff educator should have easy access to the educational resources in the system and should meet regularly with the system staff educators to share new ideas and plan educational programs. Attendance at staff education programs remains high and includes all relevant staff.

Chief Nurse (Gray Health System): The Brown VNA nurses and other clinicians should feel comfortable contacting any staff within the system and should have an easy way to get the information and answers they need. Our discharge planners and liaisons should be readily accessible to the VNA clinicians. The Brown clinicians should be invited to all our events and educational offerings.

Future Brown VNA Chief: All VNA staff should be able to contact me by phone or email or arrange appointments with me if they have concerns. Surveys from staff should indicate satisfaction.

Gray Health System HR Director: There should be new events created specifically to help the VNA staff and the Gray staff with whom they are most likely to interact to become more comfortable with each other. Intermittent surveys to staff both at Brown and Gray should indicate that they all feel part of a unified organization and are pleased to be working in the Gray Health System.

It is important to clarify that neither Brown VNA nor Gray Health System have any choice about moving further with the merger. That decision has already been made and is irreversible. At the next meeting, Sara instructs the group to use the index cards she distributes to write down what they can do to help smooth the VNA's adaptation to a new culture during the upcoming merger. She uses the My 15% approach. After everyone has had sufficient time to make their notes, Sara re-gathers the group and asks everyone to share their ideas (Box 13.4).

During a robust conversation about my 15%, everyone agrees with Natalie to have a rule that anyone who complains should also suggest solutions. Everyone promises to include this as a joint commitment. Sara conducts a pre-mortem analysis, asking everyone to consider how their plans might fail. She asks the group to think of the goal as a unified culture within the Gray Health System by the first anniversary of the merger. She asks: What does failure look like? She asks everyone to create a timeline from the point of failure looking backward to determine what might cause the plan to fail. Box 13.5 lists the common themes of the pre-mortem analysis.

Box 13.4 *My 15%*

Stakeholder	My 15%
Brown VNA chief nurse	I will meet regularly with clinicians and staff to try to prepare them for this change. I will work with our leaders and the staff educator to help people understand why the merger needs to happen and that we recognize the merging of cultures takes time I will also meet regularly with the incoming VNA chief to help him understand the VNA culture. I will establish a rule that anyone who complains about any aspect of the merger should have suggestions for resolution
Gray Health System chief nurse	I will work closely with Natalie and my staff to provide opportunities for the clinicians to get to know each other, especially those who will work together consistently, such as the discharge planners and liaisons
VNA nurse site managers	We will work with our staff to discuss what they feel they need to help them through this transition and convey that to Natalie
VNA clinicians	We will work with the other clinicians in our disciplines to help them understand why this is happening. We will try to quash any rumors and reassure them that we can all still work closely together within our own offices and see each other socially
Future VNA chief	I will spend time in each of the VNA offices trying to get to know the staff. I will try to be approachable and help people become comfortable with me before Natalie retires. I will meet with Natalie regularly to begin to understand how things are done in the VNA and how we can conduct the merger without too much change too fast
Gray Health System HR director	I will work with the VNA HR director to develop strategies to support VNA employees and the health system employees with whom they will interact most often so everyone can begin to feel comfortable with each other
VNA staff educator	I will explore ideas for books and in-service education that I can offer to our staff to help them understand what happens when two disparate organizations merge

Sara then asks everyone to discuss how to *preclude, monitor, and react* to these two themes (Boxes 13.6 and 13.7). She conducts this exercise anonymously with everyone utilizing T-W-S to think and write their thoughts on index cards. She then shares the ideas with the group without identifying who shared which idea.

Box 13.5 Common Themes of the Pre-mortem Analysis
Inefficiencies because people are unable to work together across the system.

- Poor communication between VNA staff/clinicians and system staff/clinicians.
- Unnecessary duplicate processes.
- Too many "chiefs."
- Each chief has a different way of doing things.

Perception that the VNA is a "step child" of the health system.

- VNA is located far from the system hospitals.
- VNA staff are not included in system events, meetings, or educational opportunities.
- VNA clinicians are paid differently from system clinicians.

Box 13.6 Inefficiencies
- *Preclude*: Create and ensure robust communication processes, including communicating clear and not mixed messages from administrators; analyze processes to avoid duplication.
- *Monitor*: Both the Brown and Gray administrators will closely monitor their staff, observe for problems, and handle them quickly.
- *React*: If necessary, processes will be altered to ensure excellent communication and unnecessary duplication.

Box 13.7 VNA as "Step-Child" of System
- *Preclude*: Consider relocating VNA to be closer to hospitals within the system. Create a plan for special events and educational opportunities specifically to help VNA staff adapt to change. Create ways of ensuring VNA staff have access to information about system events and educational opportunities. Analyze current pay scales for clinicians and determine whether they are consistent and equivalent between the VNA and the system and if not, explain why to VNA staff.

- *Monitor*: The clinical educators in the system and in the VNA will monitor attendance at educational events to see if Brown and Gray staff are mixing, when appropriate to the topic. The Brown and Gray chief financial officers will monitor pay scales and processes to ensure they are fair and equivalent across the system.
- *React*: If necessary, people who refuse to acknowledge and treat the VNA as part of the system will be remediated.

Sara suggests the administrators survey the VNA staff to ask them to identify behaviors that would indicate failure. By the end of this meeting, everyone appears committed to cultivating and sustaining a smooth cultural transition. Sara plans to re-gather everyone in 3 months to conduct a *second chance meeting*.

Critical Thinking Questions

1. Could Sara have added the *4 ways of seeing* method to this case? Why? why not?
2. What are other variables that need to be considered with a merger such as this?
3. Why was stakeholder analysis so important in this case?
4. Why was pre-mortem analysis appropriate to this case?

Part III

Conclusion

Conclusion

14

This book has been an attempt to illustrate an innovative approach to making better decisions. Red Teaming can improve decision-making in any setting, but we have focused specifically on nursing academe and clinical settings. It is necessary that nursing, as a profession, recognizes that it has elitist tendencies within its own ranks, and there are divisions between academic/ research environments and clinical settings. We are not a unified profession. Consequently, despite more than three million of us, we have not come as far as we had hoped with regard to entry-level education, policy, or professional status. We are unified in our commitment to the highest quality patient care, but we are not always aware of what our counterparts are doing to promote patient care because academics and researchers read different journals and attend different conferences from those of bedside nurses. These statements are generalizations, of course. However, they speak to the heart of the matter regarding why we need innovative approaches to decision-making. If the profession is not to unify and it continues to have multiple personalities, then we must have a way of making sure everyone's voice is heard. Red Teaming is the answer.

The world is never going back to a pre-internet age. Everything we say or do will forever be recorded somewhere by someone. Every action organizations take will be critiqued and responded to in real time. These facts require a new way of holding conversations, making decisions, and remaining open to changing one's mind (both at the individual and organizational level) as the future unfolds. This book has provided the tools to cope with this reality.

As you use these methods and change how you think a couple of final reminders and cautions are in order:

Change Is Hard Even when a proposed change has immediate and obvious benefits, many people will instinctively resist new ways of doing things. You must persist and convert people along the way to these new approaches. In order to do so you must always avoid acting superior or threatening the egos of those who are resistant. Keep at it, show positive results, and eventually people will come around. Do not expect overnight conversions to the Red Team way of doing things. The army has

L. Neal-Boylan, S. Rotkoff, *Innovative Decision Making in Healthcare*,
https://doi.org/10.1007/978-3-030-72648-5_14

been teaching Red Team methods for 15 years and there remain those who are skeptical and denigrate these approaches as too "touchy-feely" for the military. In the aggregate though, these approaches have been embraced at the highest level and have resulted in changes to national policy.

You Cannot Fix Toxic Leaders with Red Team Methods If you find yourself working for a toxic leader (someone who never listens, believes they are always the smartest person in the room, denigrates subordinates, and generally is a miserable person for whom to work) do NOT attempt to fix them with Red Teaming. Red Team methods such as *4 ways of seeing* may help you modify your behavior to be more successful around them, but you cannot fix the leadership shortfalls of others by using Red Team methods yourself. Leaders need to embrace these methods themselves if they want to get better at leading their organizations.

Red Teaming Takes Time All of the Red Team methods embrace some version of *think-write-share.* This takes time. Red Teaming is intended to slow the process of decision-making so that full consideration of the problem, the alternative perspectives surrounding the problem, and the divergent futures resulting from the issue or problem are considered. Therefore, you cannot Red Team everything. Many things just require an immediate response. When there is time, you may want to Red Team the organization's immediate action procedures and policies, but never attempt to do so in the middle of a crisis.

Building Diverse Thinking Takes a Conscious Effort
Diversity comes in many flavors. We tend to think of diversity in terms of race, gender identity, and ethnicity. But the great value of diversity in decision-making groups is diversity of thought. This can be achieved even in fairly homogeneous populations, but you have to invest in doing so. To be clear, it is always preferred to have a good cross section of ethnic, racial, gender identity, and age diversity on the Red Team, but in some places that is easier than in others. In some cases, the nursing staff or faculty may be dominated by women; in rural areas, these may be mostly white women. There remain ways to seek out diversity of thought even in such an apparently uniform population. Consider which nurses came from large families, which from small, who stayed locally, who went away for college, who hunts and who is a vegan, who has children, who does not…the list goes on. Diversity of thought is only limited by the imagination of the person building the Red Team. If no diversity of thinking is built into the team, little diversity of thought is likely to come out the other end.

Finally, make your own way. Remember that Red Team methods and liberating structures are ways of thinking and engaging. There is no finite list. Make up your own tools and methods as required by the circumstances of the problem, the people involved, the time available, etc. As you do, ask yourself the following questions:

• Have I created a safe environment to which people can express hard truths?
• Have I given everyone the opportunity to be heard and encouraged those who are normally quiet to participate?

- Have I separated the source of ideas from the quality of the ideas so the best ideas win?
- Have I enabled the group to understand that the plan is merely a hypothesis about the future and not a description of what must happen in the future?
- Did people feel empowered and that their time was well spent during this session?

If your answer to these questions is yes, congratulations, you have been Red Teaming no matter what the tool or method you used.

Index